UNDERSTANDING
THE CONSULTATION

UNDERSTANDING
THE CONSULTATION
Evidence, theory and practice

Tim Usherwood

OPEN UNIVERSITY PRESS
Buckingham · Philadelphia

Open University Press
Celtic Court
22 Ballmoor
Buckingham
MK18 1XW

email: enquires@openup.co.uk
world wide web: http://www.openup.co.uk

and
325 Chestnut Street
Philadelphia, PA 19106, USA

First Published 1999

A catalogue record of this book is available from the British Library

ISBN   0 335 19998 4 (pb)   0 335 19999 2 (hb)

Library of Congress Cataloging-in-Publication Data
Usherwood, Tim, 1953–
    Understanding the consultation: evidence, theory, and practice /
Tim Usherwood.
       p.   cm.
    Includes bibliographical references and index.
    ISBN 0-335-19999-2 (hbk.). – ISBN 0-335-19998-4 (pbk.)
    1. Physician and patient. 2. Patients–Psychology. I. Title.
R727.3.U83   1999
610.69′6–dc21   98-33197
                                                                        CIP

Typeset by Graphicraft Limited, Hong Kong
Printed in Great Britain by The Cromwell Press, Trowbridge

To Kate, Bo and Sam

Contents

Foreword

There are many theoretical perspectives which inform our understanding of the consultation, spanning the behavioural sciences from psychology to sociology, and including the insights of psychiatry and anthropology. This book draws these threads together and places them in the context of research evidence and the practical implications of day-to-day practice. The author is not only an experienced teacher and researcher, but also a practising clinician initially as a general practitioner near Glasgow, then in inner city Sheffield as a senior lecturer, and now in Sydney as professor of general practice.

The cornerstone of general practice is the consultation about which much has been written, but there have been few attempts to synthesize theories, evidence and practice. In doing so, this book will not only be of value to teachers and clinicians, but will also enhance the academic discipline of general practice.

David Hannay
Emeritus Professor of General Practice
University of Sheffield

Preface

General practice is the easiest discipline in medicine to practise badly, and the most difficult to do well.
(Ann Rutherford, General Practitioner, Greenock)

Towards the end of my formal training for general practice, I read two books that significantly changed my understanding of primary care medicine. They were *The Anxious Patient* (Bendix 1982) and *The Doctor–Patient Relationship* (Freeling and Harris 1984). I was enjoying the challenge of medical practice in a community setting, but I felt unskilled – unable to give any real help to patients who did not present with a clearly defined disease, and confused by many of the interpersonal processes of which I was dimly aware during consultations. Reading *The Anxious Patient* gave me the first intimation that I could offer more than just a sympathetic ear to patients who presented with emotional problems. *The Doctor–Patient Relationship* showed that it was possible to analyse a consultation and to make new sense of the interpersonal processes.

My education as a family doctor has continued since then, and I have learned further ways of responding to patients, and of understanding the dynamics of our interactions. In retrospect, I realize that I have often failed to provide patients with as effective a therapeutic response as I might. This has not always been through lack of biomedical knowledge, but also through failure to understand the process of the consultation and to act appropriately. As a trainee general practitioner, and subsequently during my career, I would have appreciated a book that described a variety of different ways of understanding the consultation, each from a different perspective, and that drew out the practical implications of these points of view. No such book has appeared. Until a better text supersedes it, I hope that others who have felt a similar need will find the present volume useful.

I have had a second reason for writing this book. Since the Second World War, general practice has developed as a distinct discipline within medicine (Bridges-Webb 1996; Usherwood *et al.* 1997; Morrell 1998). Its central role in systems of health care has been recognized in Australia, the United Kingdom and elsewhere. General practice has a number of defining characteristics, including a concern to provide anticipatory, preventive care; a focus on care of the whole person in his or her family and community context; and a preference for developing and maintaining long-term relationships as a basis for providing such care. If we are to continue the development of our discipline, I believe that we must seek constantly to define, refine and articulate the knowledge, skill and conceptual basis on which it rests. I hope that this book will make a contribution to that process.

Aim and content

I have set out in this book to examine the process of the consultation from a number of different perspectives, and to identify research evidence and theoretical insights that can usefully inform day-to-day clinical practice in the consulting room. I have therefore focused on issues that are relevant to the interaction between patient and doctor. This is not because activities outside the consulting room, such as work within the practice team, or functions relating to population health, are of lesser importance – each should complement and enhance the others – but because such external processes draw on somewhat different theoretical and practical discourses.

For a similar reason, I have concentrated on ideas and research that have implications for practice during the consultation, rather than address issues of practice organization that may change how consultations are offered. Thus, for example, I have not explored the extensive literature on how external time constraints can impact on the consultation (Davidoff 1997; Howie *et al.* 1997). This is not, however, an introduction to interpersonal communication skills; there are already a number of excellent publications that describe a skills-based approach to the clinical encounter (for example, Corney 1991; Lloyd and Bor 1996; Silverman *et al.* 1998).

Methods and acknowledgements

Once I had identified, in broad terms, the perspectives to be addressed in this book, I read or reread relevant books and articles that were already known to me, that I identified from searches of the Medline, Cochrane and ClinPSYC databases, or that were cited in the reference lists of other texts. Where possible, I have based discussion of research findings on published systematic reviews. The other books and articles that I cite are those that gave the original description of an idea, that offer a particularly good overview of an issue or related research, or that otherwise seem relevant and worth reading.

I do not claim that the statements and opinions in this book reflect unbiased interpretations of the available literature. It is inevitable that the focus of my attention, the value that I have placed on various texts, and the ways in which I have interpreted them, must reflect my own beliefs, experiences and view of the world. As a partial antidote to personal idiosyncrasy, a number of colleagues have kindly read drafts of various chapters. They are Mabel Chew, Linda Gask, David Hannay, Paul Harvey, Jenny Reath, Sharon Reid, John Spencer, Frank Sullivan and Penny Westmore. I thank them for their perceptive and critical comments, and ask for their understanding where I have been too pig-headed to heed the wisdom of their advice.

There are others who have contributed in other ways, and to whom I am also grateful. My parents lovingly supported me in my desire to study medicine, and my current family show the depth of their love and fortitude by allowing me to write about it. My patients are a constant reminder of how little I know, but gamely put up with my attempts to do better. Students and my professional and academic colleagues continue to teach me, almost on a daily basis. Jacinta Evans encouraged me to start out on this project; she and Joan Malherbe and their colleagues at Open University Press have consistently demonstrated their professionalism and support.

Outline of chapters

In the first chapter I have tried to set the context of the medical consultation by reviewing studies and theoretical understandings of how people respond to illness, and of what brings them to seek medical attention. The next five chapters are concerned directly with the process of the consultation. Chapter 2 addresses information sharing and cognitive interpersonal processes. Chapter 3 explores affective processes and the development of rapport in the patient–doctor relationship. Unconscious processes are discussed from a psychodynamic perspective in Chapter 4. Transactional analysis, a development of psychodynamic theory, is applied to the patient–doctor interaction in Chapter 5. Chapter 6 explores some of the theoretical and practical implications of examining the discourse between patient and doctor.

All illness involves family, social and psychological processes, and these provide the focus of the next three chapters. Family processes in chronic illness are reviewed in Chapter 7, and the biopsychosocial model is introduced. Emotional and psychosocial problems are discussed in Chapter 8, along with approaches to their management. Chapter 9 explores models for understanding and responding to patients who somatize their psychological distress.

Of course, any consultation represents only a brief episode in a patient's life, and in his or her relationship with the doctor. The implications of this are discussed in Chapter 10.

The chapters have been placed in what seems to be a logical order, and reference is occasionally made in one chapter to another. I have, however, tried to write each as a separate essay, so that they can be read independently if wished.

A note on the use of pronouns

It has been argued – convincingly, I think – that the use of pronouns and other words that are gender-specific both reflects and reinforces discrimination on the grounds of sex (Cameron 1985). However, I find that the constant writing of inclusive expressions such as 'he or she' can produce some very turgid text. Instead, in each chapter I have made the patient one gender and the doctor the other. I have varied the presumed genders between chapters.

Some of the examples given in the text and boxes provide an exception to this rule. All the clinical vignettes are based on real patients. I have changed many features to ensure anonymity, but the gender of each has been preserved.

I have also used the first person pronoun on occasion. The monotonous use of the passive voice in much medical and scientific writing seems to me a dubious convention. By removing the active subject from the text, it offers a pretence at objectivity that I do not believe exists. I have tried to approach the writing of this book with rigour and from a critical stance, but I want to remind you, the reader, of my presence, and hence of the ultimate contestability of all that follows.

The consultation in context

> A person *goes to the doctor with an* illness; *and returns as a*
> patient *with a* disease.
>
> (John Spencer, General Practitioner,
> Newcastle upon Tyne)

Why has this person consulted me today? Much of this book
will be concerned with processes that take place during the consultation. In this chapter, however, I will try to locate the consultation in the context of the patient's life. Why does this person
perceive herself to be ill, and why has she sought a medical
consultation at this time?

The iceberg phenomenon

We all experience bodily sensations and changes that would
be called *symptoms* if we described them to a doctor during a
medical consultation. We do not, however, seek medical advice
concerning the majority of these perceptions. In 1963 Last, a
general practitioner from Australia who was in London studying
epidemiology, published a paper in the *Lancet* on the epidemiology of disease in general practice (Last 1963; 1994). Last's paper
reported for a number of common diseases the expected pre-
valence in an average British general practice, and compared this
with the number of cases that would be known to the doctor.
For every disease there would be sufferers whose condition had
not been diagnosed. The editor of the *Lancet* coined the expression
iceberg phenomenon to denote the observation that most illness

and disease in the community is not brought to medical attention. This observation has been recognized in many subsequent studies, and remains true today.

The iceberg of illness

Last's paper described an iceberg of *disease*, which may be defined as a deviation from normal bodily structure or function. Sixteen years later, Hannay published a book in which he described a study of the iceberg of *illness*, the perception of bodily changes that may indicate disease (Hannay 1979). Over the course of a year, Hannay and his colleagues interviewed a random sample of 1344 patients registered with a health centre in Glasgow, Scotland. If the patient was a child, a parent or guardian was interviewed. The interviews included questions covering a wide range from physical, mental and behavioural symptoms. Respondents were also asked questions about social problems, health service use, sociodemographic factors, and other personal characteristics. One of the most striking findings was that only 14 per cent of those interviewed reported no physical symptoms during the preceding two weeks. The mean number of physical symptoms per person was 4.3, with a range from 0 to 25. Respiratory symptoms were by far the commonest, followed by feeling tired and generally run down. Trouble with the feet, ears and eyes, skin, varicose veins and cardiorespiratory symptoms came next.

Just over half of the respondents who reported physical symptoms in the two weeks preceding their interview had sought medical advice, 51 per cent with a general practitioner, and 5 per cent with a doctor in an emergency department or other hospital setting. It used to be argued that people would seek medical attention for symptoms once they had reached some threshold of severity, or if they caused a degree of anxiety that the individual found intolerable. However, there are findings from Hannay's study that challenge this simple model of why people consult. Respondents were asked to score their symptoms in terms of the severity of associated pain or disability, and whether or not they thought the problem was serious. Twenty-three per cent of those interviewed reported at least one physical, mental or behavioural symptom that they described as severe, or which they considered potentially serious, but for which they had not sought medical advice. On the other hand, 9 per cent of respondents reported consulting about a symptom when there was no pain or disability, and which they did not think serious. Clearly, factors other than pain, disability and perceived severity were involved in the decision to consult a doctor.

Illness behaviour and consulting behaviour

What actions do people take when they first notice symptoms? They may ignore them, of course. Cunningham-Burley interviewed a number of mothers of small children about how they dealt with their children's illnesses and symptoms. She concluded that the women developed an idea of what was normal for their child, and that this included a certain amount of 'normal illness' which they expected their children to experience (Cunningham-Burley and Irvine 1987; Cunningham-Burley and Maclean 1987). For example:

SC-B: How have the children been then, sort of health wise?
Mother: Just healthy colds, and things, you know, nothing that stops her.
                    (Cunningham-Burley and Maclean 1987: 250)

Implicit in this mother's reply is the assumption that illness is a part of everyday life, and may not require any particular response. A similar attitude was found by Blaxter and Patterson (1982) in a study of three generations of socially disadvantaged families living in Scotland. Their respondents made a distinction between normal illness and more serious illness such as cancer, heart disease and tuberculosis. Normal illnesses were common and familiar, were an expected part of life, and did not necessarily merit any action on the part of the ill person. Indeed, problems such as menopausal symptoms, and symptoms that were attributed to the wear and tear of life, were not necessarily construed as 'illness' at all.

Alternatively, a person perceiving a new symptom may conclude that some action is needed. Mechanic (1962) coined the term *illness behaviour* to denote actions taken in response to perceived symptoms. Such actions may include some kind of self-care, perhaps taking more or less exercise, going to bed early, a change in diet, or self-medication. They may also include discussion of the symptoms with another person. The particular actions that a person takes may not make a lot of sense from a medical perspective, but will be rational in the light of that person's culture, health beliefs and previous experiences (Usherwood 1990).

The process of discussing symptoms with others is important. Many people discuss their illnesses, and any new symptoms, with friends, partners or family members. This is one of the principal ways in which we all try to explain, understand and come to terms with changes in our lives. In doing so we attempt to decide what is, and what is not, significant. We compare our explanations, test and expand our understanding of the issues, explore options and decide on future actions. We are social beings, and much illness behaviour is informed by discussion with, and advice from, others (see Box 1.1).

Becoming a patient

The action of seeking medical advice is one example of illness behaviour that is frequently influenced by interaction with others. Zola (1966; 1973) interviewed over 200 patients attending outpatient clinics in two Boston hospitals. The patients he classified as either Irish American, Italian American or Anglo-Saxon Protestant American. Zola aimed to explore why they had decided to consult a doctor, and identified five major reasons (which he described as *triggers*) for doing so:

- the occurrence of an interpersonal crisis;
- perceived interference with personal relationships;
- 'sanctioning' by another person of the decision to consult a doctor;
- perceived interference with work or physical functioning;
- the setting of external time criteria.

Box 1.1   Sources of patients' knowledge of their illness

Elliott-Binns, a general practitioner in Northampton, England, reported a survey of 500 patients who attended his surgery in 1985 (Elliott-Binns 1986). He asked every fifth patient who presented with a new problem, whom they had received advice from prior to the consultation, and what advice they had received. Common sources of advice were friends, spouses, other family members, the local pharmacist, and health professionals known casually to the patient. Information was also gleaned from 'home doctor' books, television, magazines and other sources. Only 12 per cent of respondents reported obtaining no advice before consulting the doctor. The advice given included suggestions about self-medication, sometimes with home remedies, and other actions.

No doubt the detailed findings of this research would be somewhat different if the survey was repeated at a different time or in a different place. However, the implications for clinical practice are clear; it is often worth asking with whom the patient has discussed his or her illness, and what they said.

Notice that the first three triggers involve interpersonal interactions. The third, in particular, describes the situation where the ill person has discussed his or her symptoms with somebody else, and has been advised or encouraged to consult the doctor. The first two triggers were common among those patients classified by Zola as Italians. The third and fourth were commonly reported by those of Irish descent. The fourth trigger was also common among Anglo-Saxon patients. The fifth was common to all three groups; it included situations where those consulting had decided to seek medical advice if their symptoms lasted longer than some specific period or occurred more than a particular number of times (e.g. 'If I am still ill on Monday then I will call the doctor' or 'If I have one more of these turns . . .'). The fact that Zola found cultural differences in the frequencies with which the triggers were reported suggests that further reasons for consulting might be identified among patients from other cultural backgrounds. Kai (1996) interviewed parents of preschool children living in disadvantaged areas of Newcastle upon Tyne, England. He found that consulting behaviour reflected parents' fears that their child might die or be permanently harmed. The parents whom he interviewed were particularly concerned about fever, cough and the possibility of meningitis. Parents appeared to assess two factors: the perceived threat to the child and their own control over the illness. These considerations were fundamental in shaping parents' actions. Fever, for example, was perceived as offering a serious threat and its development as being outside parental control; medical advice was therefore sought at an early stage. A cold, on the other hand, being amenable to control by parental actions such as wrapping the child up, was more readily tolerated.

There is some evidence that when we first experience symptoms we try to *normalize* them. That is, we attribute them to processes that are familiar, and are thus normal to us. A example familiar to many doctors is that of the man with myocardial ischaemia, who initially puts his symptoms down to indigestion. Only later, when 'indigestion' no longer seems an adequate explanation for the symptoms, does he seek attention. Another example was reported from an interview with a woman who was thinking about consulting a doctor about backache:

> If I knew how I did it, say from lifting a bucket of coal, I wouldn't go as quick as if I didn't know where it came from.
>
> (Blaxter 1983: 59)

A significant factor that may influence whether or not a person seeks medical advice is her previous experience of health care. Little and colleagues carried out a randomized trial in which they allocated patients presenting with sore throat to one of three groups (Little *et al.* 1997). Patients in one group received an immediate prescription for an antibiotic. Patients in a second group did not receive a prescription that day, but were invited to return for a prescription if symptoms were not starting to settle after three days. Patients in the third group were not offered a prescription. There was no difference between the three groups in the proportion of patients who were better after three days, in the median duration of illness, the median number of days off work or school, or in patients' satisfaction with their care. On follow-up, however, substantially more patients in the 'immediate prescription' group thought that antibiotics were effective for sore throat, and intended visiting the doctor for future episodes. Thus a doctor's actions during a consultation may have a significant influence on the patient's future consulting behaviour.

Explanatory models and folk illnesses

Helman (1990) has suggested that when we perceive ourselves to be ill we seek answers to a variety of questions, for example:

• What has happened?
• Why has it happened? Why now?
• What will happen if I do nothing about it?
• How will it affect my family if I do nothing about it?
• What should I do about it? To whom should I turn for further help?

The answers that an individual constructs to these and other questions will reflect that person's *explanatory model* of her illness. This term was introduced by Kleinman to describe 'the notions that patients, families, and practitioners have about a specific illness episode' (Kleinman 1988: 121). The explanatory model that an individual develops for an illness episode is rooted in her more general beliefs about health and disease, but refers specifically to the one particular episode of ill health. It will reflect that person's knowledge of her current illness, her previous experiences of illness, her observations of illness in others, and so forth. Often an individual's explanatory model is evident as much in her actions as in anything that she says. Explanatory models are not fixed, but are revised and modified in the light of the ideas expressed by others, the flow of events, and the perceptions of the individual. Neither are explanatory models necessarily comprehensive and rigorously coherent; internal contradictions and inconsistencies are common, and some elements may be adhered to more strongly than others.

The doctor's explanatory model

The explanatory model that a doctor applies to a patient's illness will be informed by his training and professional experience, and may be far more explicit, organized and coherent than that of the sick person and her family. It will also be privileged in the sense that medical practitioners are accorded expert status in relation to illness, and their explanations are imbued with special authority. This does not mean that others will accept an explanation offered by the doctor as a replacement for their existing explanatory model. Rather, patients and their relatives usually try to accommodate and interpret the explanations and actions of doctors within their existing understanding of health and disease.

Folk illnesses

Sometimes the explanatory model that people apply to an illness episode reflects an understanding of the pattern of symptoms and signs which is recognized by many members of their particular culture or social group. For example, Helman (1990: 112–13) described a system of beliefs about 'colds', 'chills' and 'fevers' commonly held in a London suburb. In this belief system, colds and chills were caused by penetration of cold and damp through the skin into the body. In general, damp or rain caused cold/wet symptoms such as a 'runny nose' or 'cold in the head', while cold winds or draughts caused cold/dry conditions such as a feeling of cold, shivering and muscular aches. Colds occurred mainly above the diaphragm ('a head cold' or 'a cold in the chest', for example) while chills occurred lower down ('a bladder chill' or a 'chill on the kidneys'). Colds and chills were the result of careless behaviour, such as walking barefoot on a cold floor or sitting in a draught after a hot bath. Because of this, they tended to provoke little sympathy from others, and sufferers would often be expected to treat themselves by rest in a warm bed, eating warm food and drinking hot drinks. In contrast, fevers were caused by 'germs', 'bugs' or 'viruses' which penetrate the body by its orifices to cause a raised temperature and other symptoms. Unlike victims of colds, individuals suffering from a fever were not held to blame for their illness, and could expect care from others. The germs responsible for the fever could be flushed out by fluids, starved out by avoiding food, or killed in the body with antibiotics.

Syndromes of symptoms and signs with accompanying explanatory models that are widely recognized within a culture or community have been called *folk illnesses*. As will be clear from Helman's example, folk illnesses provide sufferers and other members of their community with an aetiological explanation, a diagnosis, an approach to prevention, and prescriptions for management. They may also have a range of symbolic meanings associated with them. A feature of many folk illnesses is that they provide members of a culture with a way of expressing, through physical symptoms, emotional distress or psychosocial disharmony (Kleinmann 1988). The presentation through physical symptoms of psychological problems is known as *somatization* and is discussed further in Chapter 9. Doctors and other health professionals need to be aware of, and learn about, the folk illnesses that are current in the community in which they work. An example is given in Box 1.2.

Box 1.2   Folk illness and somatization in Greenock

My first practice was in Greenock, near Glasgow in Scotland. It was some years before I came to understand the cultural significance of the chronic neck pain with which many patients presented. The pain and accompanying disability were very real, but also functioned as a metaphor for chronic life stresses such as unemployment or life with an abusive partner. An X-ray examination was expected, as was provision of a cervical support collar. Many patients also requested certification that they were unfit for work. 'Official' recognition of their illness, for which the collar and certificate of sickness provided tangible evidence, appeared to be helpful for the patient in tolerating what were often unresolvable long-term problems in their lives. 'Cervical spondylosis' had meanings and cultural significance among the people of Greenock that had very little to do with the radiological or pathological uses of the term.

Feeling ill and becoming sick

Awareness of symptoms, and the interpretation that one is ill, may lead to far more significant changes in behaviour and social role than those implied by the construct of illness behaviour discussed above. Talcott Parsons (1951) introduced the notion of the *sick role* to describe and explain these changes. He suggested that the sick role is defined by two rights that are enjoyed by the sick person in her relationships with others:

- The sick person is allowed exemption from normal social role responsibilities, relative to the nature and severity of the illness.
- The sick person cannot be expected to get well by an act of decision or will, and is exempted from responsibility for her illness.

These rights were seen by Parsons as conditional on two obligations:

- The sick person is expected to view being ill as inherently undesirable and to want to get well.
- The sick person is obliged to seek medical or other health care as and when appropriate, and to cooperate in the process of trying to get well.

Parsons's theory of the sick role grew out of his more general proposal that society is a system composed of a large number of interlocking smaller systems, within each of which the participants act out certain roles (Johnson 1984). He further postulated that the stability of society is threatened when its members deviate from their roles, and he viewed illness as giving rise to such a threat because of the risk that an ill person might withdraw from one or more key roles (as an employee or as a parent, for example). Parsons (1951) concluded that 'it is clear that there is a functional interest of society . . . in the minimization of illness' and he saw medical practice as 'a mechanism in the social system for coping with the illnesses of its members'. He postulated the existence of a social system comprising the patient, her doctor and others with a significant role in her life. The function of this system was twofold; to provide a mechanism for legitimizing the role of the patient within society (i.e. the sick role), and for controlling the patient's behaviour while ill. Parsons's theory of the sick role is important in that it is widely quoted and has prompted considerable debate. It has also been criticized on various grounds. It has been pointed out, for example, that parents and others may not be afforded exemption from their normal role responsibilities when ill. People with mental illness may be exhorted to 'pull themselves together', while people with HIV infection may be viewed as responsible for their ill health (Sontag 1990). It will also be clear from research into the iceberg phenomenon and illness behaviour that many ill people do not seek medical care, and there may be little or no expectation by others that they will do so. A more radical critique of the theory holds that it implies a relatively passive role for the sick person, whose actions are limited largely to seeking care and cooperating with the person who provides this. Again, the empirical evidence supports a view of the ill person as having a far more active part in defining and interpreting her illness, and acting in the light of this interpretation.

Nevertheless, Parsons's general observation remains true that consulting behaviour and other aspects of illness behaviour, which are concerned with addressing the symptoms and effects of an episode of illness, may be no more than components of more far-reaching changes in a person's behaviour patterns. Especially if illness becomes chronic or debilitating, changes in a person's social role may overshadow those aspects of her behaviour that are directly related to addressing the illness itself. Furthermore, Parsons's identification of the functions of the doctor in relation to the sick person highlights the importance of a medical consultation in legitimizing an episode of illness in the eyes of others.

Implications for care

What are the implications for the practising doctor of the empirical research and theoretical models outlined in this chapter? We have seen that many symptoms are accepted as a normal part of life, and are not necessarily interpreted as reflecting illness. Indeed, even new and unfamiliar symptoms may initially be normalized by the sufferer, their family and friends. Even when the symptomatic person is thought to be ill, she and her family may do nothing other than wait to see what happens. They are however, quite likely to talk about the illness, and the ill person may change her daily habits, self-medicate or take some other actions. Such actions will be rational in the light of the understanding that she and others have of the illness. Kleinman developed the notion of an explanatory model to describe this understanding, which will change and evolve in the light of the flow of events and conversations with others. Explanatory models are developed through a combination of experience and social interaction. As a result, a person's explanatory model of an illness will both reflect and contribute to the culture of the community of which she is a member.

It is important for doctors to develop an understanding, not just of their patients' explanatory models, but of the cultural context within which these are developed. Even when the doctor's own cultural background is similar to that of the patient, he cannot assume that they are identical. There is always the risk of misinterpreting what a patient says or does, or of behaving inappropriately oneself. Where the cultural difference is clear, then the doctor should be willing to listen, to ask questions and to learn from the patient. Family doctors should make a particular effort to learn about the cultural backgrounds of their patients.

Illness may affect our whole lives. Not only may we change our daily habits, take medication or engage in other treatments, and consult the doctor, but the whole dynamic of our interaction with others may change. Parsons's theory of the sick role is one attempt to explain these changes. Other perspectives, such as those provided by family systems theory and the biopsychosocial model, will be discussed in subsequent chapters. For the present it should be noted that a person's role within her family, at work and in other contexts may be substantially altered by illness. Awareness of these changes is important in developing an understanding of the functional impact of an episode of illness; such understanding may provide the key to explaining why an acute episode of illness evolves into chronic ill health. Again, this issue will be taken up in subsequent chapters.

When illness becomes chronic the nature of the interaction with the doctor may change. No longer does the patient attend to seek advice on the treatment and implications of an *episode* of illness. Instead, visits to the doctor become one part of the ongoing process of coping with the illness. The issue of chronic illness will also be discussed further in subsequent chapters, but for now it is important to note that many of the processes discussed in this chapter continue during chronic ill health. Thus, the sick person may discuss her illness with a wide range of people including the doctor, and will be open to other sources of information such as written material and television programmes. She will evaluate and interpret this information along with her other experiences, and in doing so will develop an increasingly sophisticated explanatory model of her illness. In both acute and chronic illness, the doctor needs to understand this model and to maintain a shared understanding with the patient as a basis for effective management.

2 Information sharing in the consultation

I take general practice to be the medical specialty of managing the interface between the complexities of the science and technology of the health care system, on the one hand, and the fears, anxieties and worries of ordinary living, on the other hand.
(Michael Tan, General Practitioner, Sydney)

The patients with whom I consulted this afternoon included a young woman complaining of dysuria and frequency, an elderly man whose Parkinsonism is progressing relentlessly, a mother concerned about her toddler whose asthma had deteriorated following an upper respiratory tract infection, and a young man trying to cope with problems at work, marital disharmony and financial difficulties. I list these because they illustrate something of the range of issues that patients may wish to discuss with the doctor, as many readers of this book will be well aware. Readers will also be aware that the presenting complaint may not reflect the patient's most pressing concerns. Furthermore, the problems that patients bring to the doctor are frequently multifactorial, including both physical and psychosocial components. The young woman was worried that she might have a sexually transmitted disease; the man with Parkinson's disease is clinically depressed, and will soon have to move from his current house as a result of his increasing disability; the mother was concerned about the prognosis of her child's asthma; and the young man presented initially with atypical chest pain.

It is the general practitioner's responsibility to address both physical and relevant psychosocial aspects of the issues that the

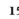

patient wishes to discuss. In order to do this, the doctor must work with the patient to:

1 understand the reasons for the patient's attendance;
2 examine other factors that affect or may affect the patient's health;
3 achieve shared definition of the issues to be addressed;
4 develop an appropriate management plan.

These tasks are similar, but not identical, to those outlined in other books on the consultation, notably those by Pendleton *et al.* (1984), Cohen-Cole (1991) and Stewart *et al.* (1995). I will elaborate on each of the tasks below. I will also discuss the role of evidence-based medicine in addressing these issues, along with evidence from research into the communication process itself. The main focus of this chapter is on the assessment and management of physical illness. In the next chapter I will discuss the role of empathy in developing rapport, and in detecting and responding to emotional distress. Later in the book, I will address approaches to helping patients with interpersonal difficulties and problems of living. Finally, I discuss the important issue of somatization in Chapter 9.

The first task – reasons for the patient's attendance

The relative importance of the tasks listed above will vary according to the circumstances of the consultation. When the patient brings a new problem for discussion with the doctor, the first task of developing an understanding of the reasons for the patient's attendance is a clear priority. In many ways this task refers to the traditional history, in which the doctor seeks from the patient an account of the problems that the latter wishes to discuss, describing the time course of symptoms and other perceptions, their effects on the patient's life, and any actions that the patient has already taken. In addition, it is important for the doctor to learn something of the patient's own ideas and beliefs about his illness, his fears and concerns, and his hopes and expectations. If the patient does not volunteer this information,

---

Box 2.1 Dangerous beliefs about the treatment of croup

Greally *et al.* (1990) reported two cases of children who were brought to hospital suffering from scald injuries. One, a 10-month-old boy, had been held over a bath half filled with boiling water. He had struggled, fallen into the bath, and sustained 12 per cent scalds. The other, a 4-year-old, had kicked over a boiling kettle and sustained superficial scalds to his hands and feet. In both cases the children were being exposed to steam in the belief that it was beneficial for the symptoms of croup.

---

then the doctor should seek it (Peppiatt 1992). Questions such as the following may be useful:

- What do you think the main problem is here?
- Have you any idea what might have caused this?
- What worries you most about this? Why does that worry you?
- How has this been affecting you?

The value of the knowledge gained will be apparent from the research discussed in Chapter 1. Without an understanding of the patient's health beliefs, the doctor will be in no position to provide an explanation that builds on the patient's existing explanatory model. At best the doctor will waste time by going over matters that the patient already knows; at worst she will fail to address potentially dangerous notions (see Box 2.1 for an example). An appreciation of the patient's fears and concerns is equally important. If these are not addressed then the patient is likely to leave the consultation feeling that the doctor has not really concerned herself with his worries. In consequence, he may be less inclined to follow the doctor's advice and may seek a further consultation elsewhere. Finally, unless the doctor knows what the patient expects from her, she will meet these expectations only by accident, if at all. Failure to address expectations is a potent cause of dissatisfaction and is a major reason why people choose not to follow medical advice (Korsch *et al.* 1968; Ley 1988).

The importance of developing an understanding of the patient's point of view is supported by the findings of a systematic review of studies of the relationship between patient–doctor interaction and patient outcome, undertaken by Stewart (1995). She concluded that outcome is improved when:

- the doctor asks about the patient's understanding of the problem, his concerns and expectations, and the impact of the problem on his life;
- the doctor asks about the patient's feelings;
- the doctor shows support and empathy for the patient;
- the patient is able to express himself fully, especially with regard to conveying feelings, opinions and information;
- the patient perceives that a full discussion of the problem has taken place.

Interestingly, a study in the United States showed that primary care doctors who exhibited these behaviours were less likely to be subject to malpractice claims, but that this finding did not apply to surgeons (Levinson *et al.* 1997).

The second task – other factors that may affect the patient's health

Good general practice is not simply reactive. Although a patient may consult about one issue, the family doctor should consider other factors that may affect the patient's health and well-being (Stott and Davis 1979). The doctor may be aware of ongoing problems that need to be reviewed. A consultation about contraception with a woman who has epilepsy might provide the doctor with an opportunity to review with the patient control of her fits, and other aspects of her disease management. Attendance by a boy with asthma, accompanied by his father whom the doctor knows to smoke, would provide the doctor with a clear opportunity to discuss the latter issue.

The second task is not concerned only with addressing problems of which the doctor is already aware. Unless there are reasons not to do so, it is a good discipline to try to address an issue of health promotion at least once during every consultation. Examples include reviewing current immunization status, performing a cervical smear, checking the blood pressure or enquiring about smoking and alcohol consumption. Of course there is rarely the time to do everything, and on occasion attempts at health promotion may be inappropriate or counter-productive. However, the option should always be considered, and a record made of any activities that are undertaken. Since the majority of people attend a general practitioner at least once a year, it is possible to cover a range of issues opportunistically during routine consultations. This is not adequate for childhood immunizations, which require a formal recall system in order to obtain population coverage. A strong case can also be made for regular recall for activities such as cervical screening, influenza immunization and so forth. The issue of preventive care in the consultation will be discussed further in Chapter 10.

The third task – definition of the issues to be addressed

The third task of the doctor is to achieve a shared definition with the patient of the issues that need to be addressed. A key step is for the doctor to summarize her understanding of the various issues back to the patient. In this way she can indicate that she has been listening to the patient's account, and can also provide the patient with the opportunity to correct or expand on her stated understanding. Summarizing need not take long. For example:

I wonder if I could check that I understand fully what you have been telling me. Ever since you were 16, you have had headaches starting above the left eye and spreading all over your head. These headaches are often preceded by zigzag lines at the edges of your vision and are accompanied by a feeling of wanting to be sick. They usually last between six and 18 hours, and seem to get better more quickly if you can lie down in a darkened room. You saw a specialist some years ago who told you that the headaches were due to migraine. Usually you get the headaches only five or six times a year, but over the last three months they have been increasing in frequency and are now occurring once or twice every week. You are missing a lot of time from work as a result. Recently you got a new boss and you have found it difficult to work with her. You wonder if your headaches are a result of this stress, but your friend told you about one of her relatives whose headaches turned out to be due to a brain tumour. You were wondering if you should have a brain scan or see a specialist about this possibility, and you would also like me to check your blood pressure. Have I got it right, or is there anything else that you think I should know?

Once the doctor has agreed with the patient a description of the relevant issues, she can undertake an appropriate physical examination and investigations. Experienced doctors tend to develop a limited number of diagnostic hypotheses while listening to the patient's account of his illness. On the other hand, unless there really is no possible alternative, they tend not to decide on a single diagnosis at this point. They use focused questions, the physical examination, and investigations, to distinguish between the possibilities that they have identified, and also to screen for rare but significant conditions (Gale and Marsden 1983; Kassirer 1989). For example, a toddler with a two-day history of cough may have a cold, early croup, otitis media or asthma, or may have inhaled a foreign body or have some other, relatively unusual, problem. Relevant focused questions would include enquiry about a history of wheeze, stridor, previous ear infections, or recent choking. Appropriate examination would include general observation of the child, estimation of the respiratory rate and temperature, examination of the ears and chest, and perhaps exclusion of nuchal rigidity. The doctor may chose to undertake a more extensive examination (taking the opportunity to auscultate the heart, for example), but the elements outlined would test the major hypotheses, while checking for signs of meningeal irritation would screen for a serious condition that must not be missed.

Clinical diagnosis in the era of evidence-based medicine

Research on the process of physical examination has demonstrated that tests vary in their reliability, sensitivity and specificity. *Reliability* measures the degree to which a test, undertaken more than once, gives the same finding. *Sensitivity* is the proportion of tests that return a positive result when an abnormality is indeed present; with a highly sensitive test, a negative finding virtually rules out an abnormality. *Specificity* is the proportion of negative results when no abnormality exists; with a highly specific test, a positive finding means that the abnormality is likely to be present. Where possible, physical examination should employ tests of maximal reliability, sensitivity and specificity in order to distinguish most effectively between relevant diagnostic hypotheses (Sackett 1992). For example, most people with ascites have a history of ankle swelling, so that such a history is a highly sensitive 'test' for ascites; if the patient denies recent ankle swelling then ascites is an unlikely cause of abdominal distension. Conversely, a fluid wave is the most specific sign for ascites, so that although many patients with ascites do not have this sign, its presence makes ascites very likely (Williams and Simel 1992). Of course, for many elements of the physical examination, the sensitivity and specificity are either not known, or are not particularly high.

Similar considerations arise in relation to investigations. These also differ in their reliability, sensitivity and specificity, and in their acceptability to the patient. It is often suggested that no investigation should be ordered unless there is a reasonable chance that the results will affect management. What constitutes a 'reasonable chance' is open to debate of course, and can provide plenty of room for negotiation within a consultation. If investigation is decided upon, and there is a choice, then it is appropriate to suggest to the patient the test or tests that will most effectively distinguish between diagnostic possibilities, and hence management options.

Once the doctor has obtained a clear account of the patient's symptoms, and has undertaken an appropriate examination and arranged relevant tests, she may be in a position to offer the patient a diagnosis. *Diagnosis* here refers to a verbal label for some recognized disorder of structure or function. In a series of studies of interactions between doctors and the parents of sick children, Korsch *et al.* (1971) demonstrated that most parents want explicit information about the nature and cause of their child's illness, including where possible, a diagnosis. A similar observation was made by Thomas (1987), a general practitioner who randomly allocated 200 consecutive patients for whom he could not make a definite diagnosis to receive either a 'positive' consultation or a 'negative' one. In positive consultations, the patient was given a firm diagnosis and told confidently that he or she would be better in a few days. In negative consultations, the patient was told 'I cannot be certain what is the matter with you' and was advised to return if he or she was not better in a few days. When surveyed two weeks later, those patients who had received a diagnosis were significantly more satisfied with the consultation than patients who had been told that the doctor was not certain what was the matter with them.

I am not suggesting that a doctor should lie when unsure of the diagnosis. However, it does seem reasonable to assume that most patients expect a clear statement of the nature and cause of their illness. It is clearly appropriate to meet this expectation honestly and frankly, and to offer an explicit diagnosis if one is available. Even if the precise cause of a patient's symptoms is not immediately apparent, the doctor may be able to offer a reasonably broad diagnostic label, or a short list of diagnostic possibilities. It may also be helpful to say if any diagnoses have been confidently excluded.

The diagnosis may raise further concerns in the patient's mind which the doctor should identify and address. It is often at this point in the consultation that the patient's expectations of care will become apparent, and again the doctor should consider asking about these. Useful questions may include:

- Can you tell me what you know about (the diagnosis)?
- Do you understand what I am telling you?
- Do you have any concerns about this?
- How would you like me to treat this?
- How have other doctors treated this problem in the past? Did that help?

In addition to providing a diagnosis, it is usually appropriate for the doctor to give a fuller explanation of her understanding of the problem and the expected prognosis. Kleinman's notion of an explanatory model was discussed in Chapter 1. The patient will have come to the consultation with ideas and concerns about his illness, and he will probably modify this explanatory model in the light of what the doctor says. However, he will not merely replace his model with that offered by the doctor. Rather, he will try to make sense of the doctor's diagnosis and explanation in the light of his understanding of the terms that the doctor uses, and of his experience of the illness to date. This interpretation may then be incorporated into the patient's explanatory model. Of course, the patient may doubt the accuracy of what the doctor tells him, in which case fewer of the doctor's ideas are likely to be incorporated in this way. Even when the patient accepts what the doctor has said, his interpretation may differ significantly from the doctor's intended meaning. The language of diagnosis is a technical one in which terms are used with consistency and precision. The same words may be understood quite differently in other contexts (think of *shock*, *chronic* or *anaemic*, for example). For these reasons it is useful for the doctor to check that the patient accepts her diagnosis as reasonable, and to enquire after his understanding of what she has just said.

The fourth task – the management plan

The development of a management plan is the phase in the consultation to which the doctor brings her understanding of pathology, therapeutics and prognosis; and the patient brings knowledge of his lifestyle, priorities and preferences. This distinction is not absolute, of course. As the doctor gets to know the patient, she will come to know something of his life, his likes and dislikes, and his view of himself and the world. The patient, particularly if his illness is chronic, may have a detailed and sophisticated understanding of his disease and its management. Although her technical knowledge is important, the key role for the doctor is facilitatory, working with the patient to develop an agreed plan.

Many writers have stressed the importance of the management plan being tailored to the particular needs, wishes and circumstances of the patient's life (Sullivan and MacNaughton 1996). In practice, such sensitivity to the patient may be the exception rather than the rule. Tuckett *et al.* (1985) undertook a study of 1470 tape-recorded consultations in general practice in the United Kingdom. They concluded that although doctors usually shared with their patients some of their reasons for their actions, doctors 'did little to encourage patients to present their views [,] . . . very rarely explored what a patient was understanding of what they said, and did not usually tailor advice and instructions to known details of the patient's life' (Tuckett *et al.* 1985: 205).

Does this matter? Is it important for the doctor to seek the patient's views on management, to explore the patient's understanding of his illness, or to tailor her advice to his needs? Stewart's (1995) review of the relationship between patient–doctor interaction and patient outcome was mentioned earlier. With respect to development of the management plan, she concluded that outcome is improved when:

- the patient is encouraged to ask questions;
- the patient is provided with clear information;
- the doctor offers emotional support;
- the doctor is willing to share decision-making;
- the doctor and patient agree about the nature of the problem and the need for follow-up.

It has to be said that the number of studies identified by Stewart was not large, and that important questions remain about the generalizability of these principles. There may be significant cultural variations in the most appropriate style for the doctor. The nature of the patient's illness may also be relevant. Research by Savage and Armstrong (1990), for example, suggested that for consultations about acute physical problems, patient satisfaction is higher if the doctor's style is directing rather than sharing. In a review of published research on shared decision-making, Charles *et al.* (1997: 683) concluded that 'while patients typically express high preferences for information about their illness and its treatment . . . their preferences for participation in treatment decision-making are much more diversely distributed'.

What about the contribution of the doctor's knowledge and understanding to this process of developing a plan? While the patient is the expert on his life, the doctor usually has more knowledge of disease and its management. Unfortunately doctors may not apply all that is currently known to the care of their patients. It is just not possible to keep up to date with all the published research that is relevant to medical care, especially in a discipline with as wide a remit as general practice. Furthermore, the human brain is not especially good at the optimal integration of a large amount of diverse, and potentially conflicting, evidence. We suffer from *bounded rationality*, the tendency to focus on a relatively small number of pieces of information, and use only these in our decision-making. It is partly to overcome this limitation that clinical practice guidelines have been developed and promoted in growing numbers.

Early clinical guidelines were consensus statements, representing the opinions of clinicians with expertise in the relevant field. However, guideline producers should nowadays attempt to overcome the obvious shortcomings of such statements through rigorous analysis and interpretation of current scientific knowledge, based on systematic review using methodologies like those developed by the Cochrane Collaboration and others (Eccles *et al.* 1998). Such evidence-based guidelines can provide the doctor with a valuable framework for discussing management options with the patient. The quality of published guidelines does vary of course, and they should never be accepted uncritically. Box 2.2 contains a list of questions to assess the quality of clinical guidelines. Even if the guidelines are of the highest possible quality, there may still be compelling reasons for a particular patient or his doctor to make choices other than those recommended (Fahey 1998; Kerridge *et al.* 1998). Such choices will, however, be informed by the best evidence current at the time when the guidelines were developed.

In future, it seems probable that interactive guidelines and other decision support resources will be increasingly available via the Internet, on computers located in clinical settings (Hovenga *et al.* 1996; Hunt *et al.* 1998). Such resources can greatly benefit the consultation, as the doctor's role shifts from that of source of

---

Box 2.2 **Questions to appraise the quality of clinical practice guidelines**

- Are the aims of the guidelines explicit? Is there a clear statement of the health problem, patients, providers and settings which the guidelines address?
- Has the process of developing the guidelines been made explicit, and was this process rigorous? In particular, was the evidence on which the guidelines are based obtained through a process of systematic review, and was it synthesized using the strongest applicable methodology (for example, meta-analysis to combine the results of multiple randomized control trials)?
- Was the process of guideline development multidisciplinary, and were both general practitioners and consumers involved?
- Do the guidelines contain statements that indicate the strength of the recommendations in the light of the research evidence?
- Was the guideline development process outcome-focused?
- Are the guidelines flexible and adaptable to varying local conditions?
- Were the guidelines developed and endorsed by authoritative bodies?
- Do the guidelines contain recommendations for evaluation and audit of the process of care?
- Were the guidelines published comparatively recently, and do they state when they will be reviewed?

---

knowledge to collaborator, working with the patient in evaluating and planning how to apply knowledge that they can both access (Del Mar and Jewell 1998).

Advising the patient

At some point during most consultations, usually towards the end, the doctor will need to offer the patient advice and guidance. This may include information about expected prognosis, plans for investigation or referral, details of a prescription or arrangements for follow-up. Ley (1988) reviewed a large number of studies of patients' recall of information provided by doctors. He concluded that patients may forget a great deal of the information that is given during a consultation. This is clearly a matter of profound concern, and it is up to the doctor to do all that she can to reduce forgetting and to maximize accuracy of recall. Techniques that Ley (1988) and others have shown to be effective include the following:

- explicit categorization – telling the patient what you are going to say before you say it;
- providing information that must be remembered first, before giving further information and advice;
- focusing only on what is important;
- giving advice that is specific rather than general – for example, 'Take the tablet just before you have supper' rather than 'Take the tablet once a day, before food';
- summarizing, stressing those points that must be remembered;
- asking the patient to repeat what they have been told, or what they are going to do, in order to check understanding;
- supplementing verbal advice with written material – this can be highly effective, but must supplement verbal advice and discussion, not replace it.

If the patient has a chronic illness such as asthma or diabetes, or presents with a number of problems that require action, then the management plan is likely to involve both short- and long-term components. Some issues – those concerned with the relief of current symptoms, for example – need to be addressed immediately. Others, such as advice on lifestyle or screening procedures, may be less urgent. Ley's (1988) studies of patient recall suggest that it can be counter-productive to address everything at once. It may be possible to agree on priorities with the patient, and deal with the various issues over a series of consultations. One of the strengths of family practice is its potential for the provision of care that is structured, proactive and continuing.

3 Empathy and rapport

Computed tomographic scans offer no compassion, and magnetic resonance imaging has no human face. Only men and women are capable of empathy.

(Howard M. Spiro 1992)

We all know doctors who, while knowledgeable and technically competent, succeed in alienating many of their patients. Conversely, there are doctors who may be less up to date in their medical knowledge, but who have a loyal following. While there is no excuse for failure to maintain technical knowledge and skills, doctors also need to display those attributes required to establish and maintain an appropriate emotional bond, or *rapport*, with patients and others. A key element in the development and maintenance of rapport is the display by the doctor of *empathy*, or emotional sensitivity, towards the patient. Of course, empathy alone is not enough. The patient also needs to feel that the doctor *respects* her, and that he is to be *trusted* in his words and actions. In this chapter I will discuss the constructs of empathy, trustworthiness and respect, and explore verbal and non-verbal ways through which the doctor can demonstrate these qualities.

Empathic understanding

The construct of empathy is an evolving one. At the beginning of the twentieth century, the German word *Einfühlung* was adopted from the discipline of aesthetics to denote interpersonal knowledge. Later, the neologism *empathy* was coined to translate the German word (Brothers 1989). These days, the term is used in a number of different ways, with somewhat different meanings implied, but the idea of emotional sensitivity is common to all.

In the clinical context, it is useful to distinguish two components in the process of responding empathetically to the patient. The first is that of developing *empathic understanding* of how the patient is feeling, and the second is that of *empathic action* to demonstrate this understanding. The two components are not independent; it is clearly not possible to act empathetically unless one has achieved a degree of empathic understanding. Furthermore, demonstration of empathy by the doctor will usually induce the patient to communicate more information about her emotional state, which the doctor can use to enhance his empathic understanding (Goldberg *et al.* 1993). Nevertheless, the distinction is useful as it provides the opportunity to consider each component separately.

Many clinicians have written about the process of developing empathic understanding. Such understanding is not merely cognitive recognition by the doctor of mood states such as anger, depression or anxiety. Our feelings are more complex than this. Even when one emotion predominates, we can normally identify others that relate to specific issues and events in our lives. As I write this paragraph I am feeling relaxed and comfortable, sitting in the sun. I also feel confident that I will eventually complete the text of this book, although I feel somewhat anxious about achieving this task by the deadline agreed with the publisher. In addition, I feel excited in anticipation of a family outing planned for tomorrow, and sad at the thought of my father's current ill health. In a useful article, Halpern (1993) has explored the notion of *emotional resonance* with the patient, and has suggested that the doctor's goal should be to seek to understand what the patient is feeling 'in a detailed, experiential way' (Halpern 1993: 162). *Detailed* understanding by the doctor implies awareness of the range and complexity of the patient's feelings, and of the issues to which they relate. To understand another's feelings in an *experiential* way does not necessarily imply sharing those feelings, but does mean seeking to comprehend what it would be like to be that person, living that person's life and feeling the way that she or he does.

As social beings, most adults have highly developed skills in sensing and interpreting the emotional processes of others. Usually we employ these skills without much in the way of conscious thought. However, it is possible to describe these skills and to develop them through practice. We sense the emotions of others through four main channels: what we hear, what we see, what we feel and what we imagine. Rogers (1975: 2) coined the expression 'listening for the feelings' to describe use of the first of these channels. Patients frequently hint verbally at their feelings during consultations (Suchman *et al.* 1997). Such hints may be quite explicit (e.g. 'I feel really fed up') or may be more tangential (e.g. 'This headache is starting to get me down'). Verbal expressions of feelings are sometimes called *verbal cues*. Often, patients' emotions are expressed more in *how* things are said than in *what* is said. It can be very instructive to listen to an audio-recording of a consultation, and to notice how the patient's voice changes as she talks about particular issues. She may sound excited as she mentions her children, anxious as she discusses a forthcoming operation, or sad when she describes how a close relative died of cancer.

Much of the time we communicate how we feel through non-verbal behaviours. These include posture, gestures, facial expressions, general appearance and observable physiological responses such as changes in respiratory rate and depth, blushing or pupil dilation. Even when we are interacting verbally, we emit a constant stream of such *non-verbal cues*. While some gestures will be conscious and intentional, much non-verbal behaviour is unconscious and reflects how we feel about the person with whom we are interacting, what is being discussed, and perhaps other issues. The expression *emotional leakage* describes the unintentional emission of non-verbal signals that are not under conscious control. Interestingly, we tend to leak different emotions in different ways: the face conveys happiness and anger best, the voice sadness and fear, and the body tension and relaxation (Argyle 1994).

Perhaps the principal way in which we communicate our emotions with conscious intent is through facial expressions. Ekman *et al.* (1972) have suggested that there are six main facial expressions, corresponding to the emotions of happiness, surprise, fear, sadness, anger, and disgust or contempt. These facial expressions seem to be much the same in all human cultures. However, culturally specific rules specify when, and to what extent, emotions may be displayed. This is clear, for example, in the different ways in which grief at the death of a loved one is expressed in different cultures. Visible non-verbal behaviour, whether or not intentionally produced, provides important cues about emotional processes but can never be decoded with absolute certainty. The lesson for the clinician is to notice these signals, and to think about their possible meanings, without making too little or too much of them.

The third channel through which we are able to sense the feelings of others is through awareness of our own feelings. There is a lot of evidence for *emotional contagion*, some primitive process through which we 'catch each other's emotions' (Argyle 1994: 45). Listening to a depressed patient, we may ourselves begin to feel frustrated and overwhelmed; talking with someone who is excited about a forthcoming event, we may begin to feel excited about it too. Several different mechanisms may account for this process (Brothers 1989), but the relevance for the clinician is that it is worth noticing and paying attention to one's own feelings during the consultation. Self-knowledge is needed here. I may be feeling uncomfortable and defensive because I neglected to test for glycosuria in an earlier patient who mentioned a recent history of weight loss, or because I had an argument with a colleague. Alternatively, I may be reacting to the current patient's unexpressed anger at being kept waiting because I am running late.

Finally, a valuable sense of how a patient feels may be gained from imagining oneself in that person's shoes. I am a middle-aged, middle-class, male professional, but I can try to understand some of the feelings of frustration, fear, anger, anxiety, resignation and contempt experienced by a young woman living in poor-quality housing with an abusive partner who misuses alcohol and has recently lost his job. I can attempt this by imagining how I might feel if I were living in her situation and facing her options in life.

Of course, sensing cues and imaginatively guessing at the emotional processes of another are not the same as accurately knowing how that person is feeling. Such knowledge requires two further steps: interpretation of the available sensory and imaginative data, and checking back with the patient. The basic requirement for the process of interpretation is an attitude of free-floating curiosity (Halpern 1993). This is not the curiosity of the biochemist seeking to understand a derangement of metabolism, but that of one human being seeking to understand and engage with another. As such, it must not get in the way of listening to the patient in the here and now of the consultation. However, in much the same way as it is possible to listen for details about the site, radiation, quality, intensity and time course of pain while attending to the patient's story without interruption, so it is possible to maintain a level of curiosity about the patient's feelings without becoming distracted by them. If brought more fully into consciousness, such curiosity might give rise to questions such as 'I wonder why the patient said that, in that way, just now? I wonder why she has not told me about her relationship with her partner? I wonder why I feel this way at this moment? I wonder what it would be like to be this person?'

Empathic action

However competent the doctor becomes in his interpretation of the patient's verbal and non-verbal cues, and of his own emotional and imaginative responses to the patient and her story, his ideas about her feelings can remain only hypotheses until he has checked them out with the patient herself. Such checking out, described here as *empathic action*, has two purposes. The first is to help the doctor confirm and refine his empathic understanding. The second is to communicate this understanding to the patient. Clearly, if the doctor is very wrong in his interpretation of how the patient is feeling, then communication of this will do little to enhance their relationship. It follows that unless the doctor is very sure of his ground, demonstrations of empathy are best offered in a tentative manner. A number of examples are given in the next paragraph and in Box 3.1. On the other hand, if the doctor's demonstration of empathy is accurate and appropriate then the patient is likely to confirm this in two ways. The first is some kind of verbal or non-verbal indication that the doctor is right. The patient may nod, say something like 'That's right' or indicate agreement in some other

---

Box 3.1   Further examples of empathic statements

Observations on experience
You've really been through a lot.
That's a lot of problems to face all at once.
You must have felt very frightened when that happened.

Observations on behaviour
You must have been feeling very angry to do that.
That must have been very difficult to do.
You don't seem entirely happy about doing that.

Self-disclosure by the doctor
It makes me sad to hear that.
I feel quite confused; I wonder if you do as well?

Statements of 'I . . . you . . .' form
I can see that it's very difficult for you to talk about this.
I can understand that you must find that very painful.

---

way. Second, the patient will probably provide further information about her feelings and problems (Hobson 1985; Egan 1994).

Perhaps the simplest way of demonstrating empathy is through the verbal acknowledgement of a verbal or non-verbal cue: 'You look upset' or 'You mentioned that you feel fed up', for example. Empathic observations can be offered more tentatively: 'I wonder if you feel sad'. Alternatively, the doctor can ask a question: 'Do you feel sad about that?' If the doctor is responding to the patient's description of an event then he may be able to imagine how she felt: 'You must have felt very scared when the surgeon told you that he thought it was breast cancer' or 'It is very frightening to see your child so ill, and not be able to do anything about it'. More elaborate expressions of empathy acknowledge underlying experiences and behaviours, as well as the feelings themselves. Examples are provided in Box 3.1.

Not all empathic action is verbal, of course. Sometimes touch or other actions are an appropriate way of demonstrating empathic understanding, although they are more open to misinterpretation by the patient. Also useful is the concept of *matching* described by Neighbour (1987). He depicts this in the following terms:

> You intentionally adjust your own behaviour so that it more nearly resembles those aspects of the patient's which you have particularly noticed. You might match your delivery and speech . . . to the patient's, and/or your voice delivery, and/ or your posture and gestures, so that a third party observing the pair of you would be struck by the similarities.
> (Neighbour 1987: 142)

Neighbour is not suggesting here that doctors should mimic their patients; to do so would clearly destroy rapport, perhaps irrevocably. Rather he is suggesting matching of the most salient features of the patient's behaviour, motivated by a genuine concern to put the other person at ease. He makes the important observation that while matching of behaviour is clearly observable between two people who have a high level of rapport (think of a couple at a party who are obviously getting on well together), the process also works the other way. That is, intentional, unobtrusive matching of behaviour can enhance rapport (Lankton 1980).

The uses of empathy

I started this chapter by suggesting that display of empathic understanding by the doctor is important for the development of rapport. However, the uses of empathy are not limited to this function. Egan (1994) and Halpern (1993) have identified further uses for empathic understanding. First, awareness by the doctor of how the patient may be feeling as she tells her story can provide an important guide in asking additional questions, and in behaving in ways that will invite rather than discourage further communication. It is well known, of course, that a patient may present with one problem when it is another that is really troubling her. An empathic sense that something else is wrong may be the doctor's first clue (see Box 3.2 for an example). Second, empathic sensitivity can also help the doctor understand the meaning behind the words which the patient uses to describe her symptoms. A patient with profound anaemia and a

---

Box 3.2   A 'ticket of admission'

A 54-year-old man with diagnosed hypertension presented for 'a blood pressure check'. The doctor sensed that the patient was concerned about something, and asked: 'Is there anything else worrying you?' The patient responded: 'Can those blood pressure tablets make you impotent?'

---

patient suffering depression may both complain of tiredness. However, the empathic clinician may sense a quite different emotional quality to the complaint of each patient. Third, empathic understanding of the health values and the meaning of illness to the patient and her family can provide a guide to treatment, and to the formulation of a management plan that is acceptable to the patient. As Halpern points out, it is our emotions that determine what is important to us. Finally, it has been suggested that the demonstration of accurate empathy can be directly therapeutic for the emotionally distressed patient (Rogers 1957). The research evidence is, however, conflicting on this issue (Barkham 1988).

So far I have discussed the development of empathic understanding and its demonstration through empathic action as if these are in a linear sequence, the one following the other. However, as I suggested earlier, one of the uses of empathic action is to help the doctor test and deepen his empathic understanding. In doing so he is also likely to help the patient deepen her own understanding of her feelings and of her emotional responses to illness and other events in her life. Empathic understanding is more accurately seen as a mutual understanding that is jointly developed by patient and doctor working together. It is the doctor's responsibility to facilitate this process.

Empathy and intimacy

Expressions of empathy, and the sharing of personal thoughts and feelings, may lead rapidly to feelings of warmth and closeness.

However, closeness and intimacy are not goals in themselves. Some patients feel threatened by naming and discussion of feelings, and it is generally appropriate to respect this and to deal instead in experiences and behaviours. At other times, an early and accurate expression of empathy may engender a sense of intimacy before the patient has learned that she can trust the doctor. This can also feel threatening to the patient. Demonstrations of empathy early in the consultation should be offered with sensitivity and care.

Conversely, a deep sense of connectedness with the patient is experienced during some consultations. These moments may occur when the doctor and patient have established a firm and trusting relationship, and the doctor makes a particularly accurate empathic statement, or when the patient discloses some particularly personal aspect of his or her life. Matthews *et al.* (1993: 973) have written about 'the powerful and mutual experiences of shared understanding that characterize these moments' and suggest that they are often marked by a physiological reaction such as gooseflesh or a chill; by an immediacy of awareness of the patient's situation; by a sense of being part of a larger whole; and by a lingering feeling of joy, peacefulness or awe.

Cyril Gill, one of the early Balint group members, has pointed out that such occasions are characterized by spontaneous mutual awareness of something that is important to the patient (Gill 1973). Enid Balint went further to suggest that

> the flash of understanding . . . may expose the tip of an iceberg, or the heat of a fiery cauldron, which, perhaps, over the weeks or months or years can gradually be explored either by the patient and doctor together or by the patient alone, and the patient then finds he can make more use of himself and of his environment.
>
> (E. Balint 1973: 21)

Such a moment of insight may provide the first evidence for both doctor and patient of significant psychosocial issues in relation to what was previously seen as a predominantly physical problem.

Whether or not the patient and doctor experience some moment of profound closeness and mutual understanding, emotional intimacy brings several potential dangers to the relationship (Matthews *et al.* 1993). The first is that of intensifying the patient's dependence on the doctor. We probably never completely extinguish the wish to be thoroughly cared for by an omnipotent parent. When we are sick we tend to regress to a more childlike state, and the discovery that the doctor is capable of deep understanding and empathy may exacerbate the regression. The second danger is that associated with the development of sexual feelings in the doctor or patient. Doctors do sometimes feel sexually attracted towards their patients, but acting on those feelings is never appropriate and is extremely likely to bring harm to the patient (Rutter 1995). It is a mistake to deny such feelings to oneself, but it is important to deal with them elsewhere, perhaps through discussion with a trusted colleague.

Patients occasionally express sexual feelings towards their doctors, but for the doctor to reciprocate in any way is once again fraught with the risk of causing harm. Sexual overtures from a patient should not be ignored, but should be responded to in a firm and non-judgemental manner. If they persist, then it is useful to discuss the matter with a colleague in the practice. Ultimately, it may be necessary to advise the patient to attend another doctor (Golden and Brennan 1995). Medical regulatory bodies such as the General Medical Council in the United Kingdom, and boards and tribunals in other jurisdictions, rightly regard any sexual activity between doctor and patient as indicative of professional misconduct, whether or not the patient expressed consent or even initiated the activity.

The final challenge for the doctor is that of experiencing the pain of the patient. Empathic understanding is, by definition, experiential, and if the patient's distress resonates in some way with our own lives, fears or unresolved issues, then we may feel overwhelmed by the experience and find ourselves no longer able to offer the help that we should. Partial identification with the patient occurs for all doctors on occasion, and once again discussion with a trusted colleague is important. Often another doctor in the practice can provide appropriate support, but many doctors find co-counselling useful, or even professional supervision by a suitably qualified counsellor or psychotherapist. Affirming relationships and sources of meaning outside medicine are also important.

Trustworthiness and respect for the patient

At the start of this chapter I suggested that while empathy is necessary for the development and maintenance of rapport within the patient–doctor relationship, it is not sufficient on its own. Demonstration by the doctor of trustworthiness, and of respect for the patient as an individual, are also necessary.

Trustworthiness is an attribute expected of all professionals, and is underpinned by professional codes of ethics. Respect for confidentiality, and the obligation to place the patient's interests ahead of one's own, are examples of codified injunctions to behave in a trustworthy manner. The growth of trust between an individual doctor and patient takes time, and depends on the doctor acting with integrity, competence, consistency and commitment. *Integrity* depends on intellectual and emotional honesty, with oneself as well as the patient. *Competence* reflects clinical ability, including awareness of the limits of that ability, and hence knowledge of when to refer to or seek advice from a colleague. *Consistency* implies congruence between the doctor's words, actions and other non-verbal behaviour. Finally, *commitment* means that the doctor's actions are in the best interests of the patient, and reflect the open-ended nature of the relationship in primary care. Further consultations may occur with any patient, and the patient–doctor relationship ends only with the death of one or the other. Furthermore, the patient is free to bring any issues or concerns to the consultation, and can reasonably expect the general practitioner to respond in a committed and appropriate manner.

The third necessary condition for rapport is demonstration by the doctor of non-judgemental *respect* for the patient – what Rogers (1957) and others have called 'unconditional positive regard'. Respect means prizing the patient simply because she or he is human. When consulting with a person convicted of child abuse, I may abhor his past actions, but I must still acknowledge his value as a human being and the needs and rights that flow from this. Such respect is more than an attitude of mind; it implies an active attempt to address these rights. All doctors feel dislike for some patients (Mathers *et al.* 1995). Active respect means overcoming that dislike in order to treat the patient to the best of one's ability (Groves 1978).

In an article provocatively entitled 'When Balinting is Mind-rape', Zigmond (1978) pointed out that as a doctor becomes more aware of psychosocial issues, and more sensitive to emotional cues, he may unthinkingly start to use this awareness in a way that is abusive and potentially damaging for the patient. A patient may be emotionally distressed when she consults the doctor, but this does not mean that she wishes to discuss the underlying issues, which may be of no relevance to the problems that she actually wants addressed. Zigmond suggests that the stereotypical complaint 'My doctor is always in such a rush and doesn't seem to listen' may be replaced with a new one: 'My doctor is always trying to listen to things I don't want to tell him.' He goes on to point out that the asymmetry of power in the patient–doctor relationship can make the patient very vulnerable to psychic intrusion by the doctor. The solution that he proposes is to respect the patient's right to privacy, and to seek her explicit consent when exploring painful issues: 'Do you want to talk about that' for example, or 'Don't tell me unless you are ready'. Checking with the patient in this way demonstrates both respect and trustworthiness on the part of the doctor.

Transcultural consulting

In many consultations, patients and doctors have cultural backgrounds that are quite distinct from each other. Rapport may be more difficult to establish and maintain in transcultural consultations for a number of reasons. There may be a history of oppression and racist behaviour by people of one culture towards people of the other. Aspects of the practice in which the consultation occurs (such as an appointment system) may not be culturally appropriate for the patient. There may be cultural norms for the patient that dictate what behaviour is acceptable from the doctor, and what actions are befitting for the patient. The doctor may offend or embarrass the patient by inadvertently transgressing these norms. These norms may differ according to the gender of the patient and of the doctor. There may also be cultural limitations on what can be discussed with the doctor. Again, these limitations may differ with gender. Finally, cultural differences in the words and metaphors used to describe distress, and in the non-verbal display of emotion, and may make it difficult for the doctor to interpret the patient's communications.

For these reasons, doctors working with patients from different cultural backgrounds need to learn as much as they can about those cultures, the ways in which illness and disease are understood within them, the norms of behaviour that are expected of doctors, the courtesies and the taboos. An interesting book by Qureshi (1994) provides a useful reference with information about these issues in relation to many different cultures, but people vary, and perhaps the most useful sources of learning for family practitioners are their patients.

4 Psychodynamic insights

If you ask questions you get answers – and hardly anything else.

(Michael Balint 1986: 133)

A junior hospital doctor consulted her general practitioner several times over the course of three months with a series of apparently unrelated, self-limiting conditions. When the general practitioner eventually commented on this, the young woman sat deep in thought for several seconds and then started to cry. It transpired that she was working on an oncology ward. Her father, to whom she had been very close, had died from cancer while she was at medical school. The sufferings of her patients reminded her of the suffering of her father, and the inevitable death of some patients recalled many of the feelings that she had experienced when her father died. In order to cope and to keep working, she pushed these thoughts and feelings out of conscious awareness. However, she began to feel increasingly unhappy and to lose confidence in herself and in her choice of career. She also became less confident about recognizing the self-limiting nature of many symptoms, which was probably one reason for her increased rate of consulting. As the general practitioner continued his conversation with her, he began to wonder whether she was also using him to replace the missing father in her life. Simultaneously, he became aware of paternal feelings towards her, as if she were one of his daughters, although the general practitioner's real daughters were more than ten years younger than the patient.

This account illustrates a number of important psychological processes, or *dynamics*, including the defence of repression, return of repressed material, overdetermination of behaviour, transference and counter-transference, all of which will be discussed below. The first person to provide a coherent theory of psychodynamic processes was, of course, Sigmund Freud. The collected writings of Freud run into many volumes, and a vast amount has since been written about psychodynamic theory and its clinical application. In this chapter I will not attempt a review of the whole theory but will discuss a number of ideas and insights from the theory that are particularly relevant to primary medical care. I will also outline the contributions that the psychotherapists Michael and Enid Balint made to understanding the process of general practice.

Transference and counter-transference

Transference is a key concept in psychodynamic theory, and refers to projection on to the therapist by the client of feelings, ideas and other attributes which derive from previous figures in the latter's life (Storr 1989). Freudian therapists act in a way that is intended to maximize transference by the client (Malan 1995), but the process of transference probably occurs in all relationships, including those between patient and doctor. It is suggested that from our very earliest relationships, which are usually with our parents, we develop feelings and beliefs about others which then colour our subsequent relationships. Occasionally this transference may be particularly intense and can interfere with the development of a relationship that reflects the reality of the here and now of the individuals concerned. Ideally, the patient–doctor relationship in general practice is a working alliance, to which both the patient and the doctor bring their knowledge, ideas and concerns, and in which they work together to address the patient's problems (see Chapter 2). The development of significant transference will inhibit the development of an effective relationship because much of the patient's behaviour, verbal and otherwise, will reflect his response to the attributes that he has projected on to the doctor rather than the reality of their need to work together. An example is given in Box 4.1.

Box 4.1   Transference in the patient–doctor relationship

A man in his late twenties consulted his male general practitioner, seeking help with headaches and a growing feeling that he could no longer cope with the responsibilities of his job. The headaches had the characteristics of tension-type headaches, and on physical examination the doctor found nothing to suggest an alternative diagnosis. When asked, the patient readily agreed that the headaches were probably related to stress at work and in other areas of his life. When asked to expand on the latter, the patient explained that his older brother, to whom he was very close, was seriously ill with testicular cancer. The doctor spent some time listening to the patient, discussing his feelings and his fears about his own health, and exploring ways in which he could let his brother know how much he meant to him. The doctor also examined the patient's testes and advised regular testicular self-examination. Finally, he invited the patient to return for review.

The patient returned about two weeks later and reported that he and his brother had spent a long evening talking about their childhood together, their mutual family, and their feelings for each other. Subsequently the patient's headaches had become much less intense, and he was coping better at work. Rather than attribute these developments to his own actions, the patient praised the doctor for what he had done, and expressed his admiration for the doctor's depth of understanding and competence. The doctor, who knew his limitations only too well, felt somewhat embarrassed at the idolization. However, he had already learned from the patient that the latter had virtually worshipped his brother when younger, and before his illness had continued looking to him for advice and guidance. When they were children, the two boys had idolized their father, who was in the Royal Navy and was away at sea for months at a time. The doctor realized that the patient was projecting on to him feelings from his relationship with his brother, feelings that had their origin in his relationship with his father.

Of course, it is not just the patient who may introduce into the consultation issues from other relationships. The doctor may do likewise, particularly where some characteristic of the patient recalls some other person of significance in her life. Since Freud, this process has been called *counter-transference*, but the intrapsychic processes are the same as those that lead to transference. Counter-transference projections may be wholly unconscious, or the doctor may be partly aware of them. Unconscious counter-transference is, of course, potentially extremely dangerous for both parties as the doctor does not relate to the patient who is in front of her, but to a composite of that person and her unconscious projections. More often, the doctor is partly aware of her counter-transference in the form of unexpected feelings towards the patient. Counter-transference feelings can be extremely powerful, and are often quite elemental – lust, fear or hate, for example. Many so-called 'heartsink' patients may be suffering from counter-transference by their doctors (Groves 1978; Mathers *et al.* 1995).

Transference and counter-transference do not just happen. They are processes that are allowed to develop, and the doctor can take steps to modify them. She may, for example, become aware of feelings in herself that do not reflect empathic understanding of the patient, but rather some other relationship in her life. She can then seek to deal with those feelings in some way that does not intrude in her relationship with the patient. It is often most helpful to discuss such feelings with a trusted friend, colleague or partner. Some doctors find regular professional supervision by an experienced psychotherapist very beneficial.

Illness and the unconscious

I have already alluded to unconscious processes in this chapter. It is useful to distinguish between what is conscious, what is pre-conscious, and what is unconscious. Conscious thoughts and feelings are those of which we are aware. Pre-conscious processes are those of which we are not aware, but which we can bring into conscious awareness. Much verbal and non-verbal behaviour cannot, however, be adequately understood in terms of thoughts that are fully or potentially conscious; hence the need to postulate unconscious mental processes. Unconscious processes cannot be accessed directly by the individual, but must be inferred from behaviours and from conscious thoughts and feelings.

The demarcation between the pre-conscious and the unconscious is not absolute, and what cannot be consciously accessed today may become accessible in the future. Conversely, mental processes that in some way threaten the integrity of the personality may be *repressed*, which means that they are consigned to the unconscious; the individual not only forgets, but also forgets that he has forgotten (Laing 1971). The mechanism of repression can provide an important defence against being emotionally overwhelmed, perhaps by the feelings associated with the memory of some dreadful experience. Repression is probably never complete, however, and repressed material tends to re-emerge in disguised form. The young doctor's growing unhappiness and loss of confidence in the example at the start of this chapter is one instance of this process. Another, sadly familiar in clinical practice, is seen in the plethora of psychological symptoms that may be experienced by survivors of sexual abuse (Mullen *et al.* 1993).

The notion of unconscious processes often helps to make sense of how people respond to illness in their lives. One person with whiplash injury to the neck, for example, may recover fully and return to work within a few days. Another, with an apparently similar injury and in similar socioeconomic circumstances, may become a chronic invalid and stay off work for months. Although the patient may be suspected of malingering, which is a conscious act, this is rarely the case (Evans 1992). Such behaviour is often better understood in terms of unconscious processes. In particular, Freud's idea of primary and secondary gains can be helpful. Freud suggested that some symptoms arise, or are perpetuated, because they bring benefits to the patient. *Primary gain*, in psychodynamic theory, relates to neurotic symptoms, and the way in which they provide relief from anxiety and internal conflict. For example, a person with an obsessive trait might check and recheck that the front door is locked when he leaves the house. The primary gain of this behaviour is reduction in nagging worries about security.

Secondary gains, on the other hand, are those personal advantages that illness offers to the patient in his interactions with
others. They may arise from any symptoms, not merely those of
a neurotic nature. The patient who takes to his bed following an
acute back sprain may, for example, be avoiding interpersonal
conflict at home or at work. Rycroft (1995) has pointed out that
members of the patient's family tend to be acutely aware of the
secondary gains of symptoms, but oblivious to primary gain.

Some implications for practice

A number of clear implications arise for clinical practice. An
important principle is that no aspect of a patient's behaviour is
random, although the clinician may never fully understand the
reasons for it. As a corollary, much behaviour is *overdetermined*
(Malan 1995). That is to say, it can be explained in a number of
different ways. To return to the example of the patient who
develops chronic functional impairment following a back sprain,
he may be avoiding interpersonal conflict at work, and may also
be avoiding some of the demands of family life. He may suspect
that the doctors are not being entirely honest with him in the
explanations that they give, and may believe that he needs to
demonstrate the extent of his disability in order to obtain their
full attention. This belief might reflect a story that he has heard
about a man with back pain whose correct diagnosis of prostatic
metastases was delayed. It might also reflect his experiences as a
child, with parents who ignored illness in their offspring unless
the manifestations were unavoidable. Finally, the patient may
be depressed, with his back pain and disability both reflecting
and contributing to his depression.

The clinician must be aware of the potentially multifactorial
causes of illness and illness behaviour. She must listen for these
in the patient's story, must look for opportunities to intervene
at various levels, and should reflect constantly on the implications of her behaviour for the outcome of the patient's illness.
To continue with the example above, the doctor should seek
to understand and respond in detail to the patient's beliefs and
fears about his illness; she must engage with the patient collabor-
atively, as another adult, rather than as an aloof parent; she

should screen for, and if necessary treat, any accompanying depression; and, where possible, she should avoid reinforcing any secondary gain from the patient's illness. She must also accept that while disease is often relatively easy to treat, the multifactorial aetiology of illness makes it much harder to intervene effectively.

Clear boundaries are important in the patient–doctor relationship. Boundaries define the limits of acceptable behaviour for both parties. Appropriate boundaries tend to inhibit the development of inappropriate feelings and behaviours, perhaps by providing a constraint on unconscious fantasies. In many consultations, patient and doctor share a tacit understanding of these limits which do not require further elaboration. With some patients the limits need to be defined more explicitly. The ultimate in boundary setting is for the doctor to terminate her relationship with the patient, and to advise him to consult another doctor within the practice, or to attend a different practice. This step is occasionally necessary when erotic or other inappropriate feelings intrude into the professional relationship and cannot be resolved or contained in any other way (Golden and Brennan 1995).

Contributions of Michael and Enid Balint

No discussion of psychodynamic theory in relation to general practice would be complete without mention of the work of Michael and Enid Balint. The Balints were psychotherapists at the Tavistock Clinic in London. From 1950 until the early 1970s they conducted regular supervision sessions for groups of general practitioners. The overall aim of the groups was 'examination of the ever-changing doctor–patient relationship, i.e. the study of the pharmacology of the drug "doctor"' (Balint 1986: 4). Both the Balints and the doctors who participated in the Workshop, as the groups became known, recognized that patients regularly present to general practitioners with psychological problems, but that these problems are often disguised rather than overt. The groups were intended to have both training and research functions. The validity of Balint groups (as they are now known) as an approach to postgraduate training is somewhat controversial, and although strong arguments have been presented for their value (Elder 1996), relatively few such groups continue today. Furthermore, many so-called 'Balint groups' appear to have departed significantly from the process outlined by Enid and Michael Balint themselves (Scheingold 1988).

Whatever the educational legacy of the Balint seminars, the research findings remain of considerable interest. Michael Balint's book *The Doctor, His Patient and the Illness* (Balint 1986) and the collection of essays *Six Minutes for the Patient* edited by Enid Balint and JS Norell (1973) are classics of general practice literature. Enid Balint's account of the 'flash technique' was mentioned in Chapter 3. Here I will outline Michael Balint's analysis of the interaction between patient and doctor, including his theory of the doctor's apostolic function, and the problem of collusion between doctor and patient. In Chapter 9 I will discuss Balint's account of collusion between doctors.

The patient's offers and the doctor's responses

Michael Balint suggested that the patient starts the consultation by offering one or more problems and issues to the doctor. The doctor responds to these offers, indicating her acceptance or rejection of them, until some kind of compromise is worked out. In consequence, while the matters that are discussed in the consultation reflect the problems presented by the patient, they include only those aspects that the doctor indicates are allowable. Balint pointed out that it may well be appropriate for the doctor to constrain the topics that are addressed in the consultation, in order to focus on those that are amenable to management within a medical setting. He described the thoughtful and sensitive use of *selective attention* and *selective neglect* in responding to the patient's utterances as a technique for achieving this constraint (M. Balint 1973). However, he and his colleagues in the Workshop observed that the constraints imposed by doctors were often applied without much in the way of conscious thought, and Balint coined the term *apostolic function* to describe the doctor's unconscious attempts to control the patient's behaviour (Balint 1986). He chose the term 'apostolic' to indicate that it was almost as if every doctor had revealed knowledge of what was right and what was wrong for patients to expect and to endure, and further, as if he had a sacred duty to convert to his faith all the ignorant and unbelieving among his patients.

(Balint 1986: 216)

Although I cannot help feeling that Balint overstated the case here, there is no doubt that we all respond unthinkingly to our patients on occasion, and in doing so control their behaviour within the consultation. Balint's principal explanation for such actions, which I do find convincing, is that doctors tend to steer the consultation away from topics about which they feel uncomfortable. One potent source of discomfort is when the patient tries to raise psychosocial issues that in some way reflect problems in the doctor's personal life. The doctor with a seriously ill child, for example, may find it very painful to discuss a similar crisis in the life of a patient. A doctor who tends to overuse alcohol may be reluctant to engage in discussion about a patient's excess alcohol intake.

Collusion in the consultation

The second example given above, in which both patient and doctor avoid discussing an issue that is relevant to the patient's health, illustrates a process that Balint (1986) described as *collusion*. Such avoidance may, of course, reflect a conscious decision by both parties. More often, it reflects an unconscious defence on the part of each individual. The doctor may avoid a particular topic that she finds threatening, or may respond only to those offers by the patient which she feels comfortable to address. The patient may not wish to threaten his relationship with the doctor, may not link his symptoms to the avoided issue, or may collude for other reasons (see Box 4.2).

Clearly, the doctor needs to be aware of the effects of her verbal and other responses to the patient's offers in shaping the way in which his illness is defined in the consultation. On the one hand, selective attention and selective neglect, thoughtfully and sensitively employed, can focus the consultation on those

---

Box 4.2 Collusion between doctor and patient

An experienced general practitioner was consulted
frequently over a period of months by a woman to whom
he felt attracted, and who was of a similar age to himself.
At each consultation the patient complained of symptoms
of oesophageal reflux. Endoscopy had shown only mild
inflammation at the lower end of the oesophagus, but her
symptoms failed to respond to a range of treatments. During
one consultation, as the doctor was again asking about
exacerbating and relieving factors, the patient mentioned
that her symptoms were particularly troublesome during
sexual intercourse. Only then did the doctor realize that
he had been vaguely aware of difficulties in the patient's
marriage, and asked her about this relationship. The patient
confirmed that there were problems, and the conversation
moved on to discuss these.

On reflection, the doctor realized that he had
subconsciously been avoiding the topic of the patient's
marriage, in part, at least, because he had been repressing
his own sexual attraction towards her. He also wondered
if the patient's oesophageal reflux had brought her the
secondary gain of avoiding intercourse with her husband,
and if her frequent consultations had served the purpose of
legitimizing the symptoms. The patient continued to consult
the general practitioner, although less frequently, and she
reported that her oesophageal symptoms were much
reduced.

---

issues that are amenable to management within a medical setting.
On the other hand, the doctor must beware of unconsciously
steering the conversation away from relevant matters that she
happens to find personally threatening or uncomfortable. She
must be particularly careful of colluding with the patient in
avoiding significant topics. Such collusion can go on for months
or years, becoming a dominant feature of the patient–doctor
relationship, and significantly constraining the issues that either
party can raise.

5 The transactional perspective

True knowledge is to know how to act rather than to know words.

(Eric Berne in Stewart 1992: 4)

Psychodynamic theory is concerned essentially with the intra-psychic processes of individuals. Constructs such as transference, counter-transference and collusion can certainly throw light on some interpersonal processes, but the classical theory does not provide a complete account of relationships between people. During the 1950s, Eric Berne, a North American psychiatrist who had trained in Freudian psychoanalysis, began the development of an alternative theory which does claim to provide such an account (Berne 1961; 1964; 1972). *Transactional analysis,* as the theory is known, provides a useful model for understanding many aspects of interactions in the medical consultation (Freeling and Harris 1984). In this chapter I will outline the theory and discuss its implications.

Ego states and the analysis of interactions

All of us are aware that, when interacting with others, we may behave in a parental fashion, in an adult manner, or in a child-like way. Berne suggested that at any moment in time, a person who is interacting with others will always be exhibiting one of these three modes of behaviour, which he called *ego states* and referred to colloquially as Parent, Adult and Child. An Adult ego

---

Box 5.1   Two friends at a party

John: Would you pass over the packet of cigarettes? (Adult)
Jane: You know you shouldn't smoke. (Parent)
John: Do you think the evidence about passive smoking is
        convincing? (Adult)
Jane: Yes, I do. (Adult)
John: I know that I should stop. (Adult) But it is so hard,
        you know. (?Child)
Jane: I have never smoked a cigarette – I have often
        wondered what it is like. (Child)
John: Don't you start. (Parent)

---

state is typified by autonomy and orientation to the current
reality. The other two ego states have their origins in the individual's past. The feelings and behaviours of a Parent ego state
are derived from parental figures, and are typically nurturing or
controlling. A Child ego state reflects the feelings and behaviours of the individual's own childhood, and is often creative and
playful but may also be clinging and dependent. During spontaneous social interaction, most people exhibit shifts from one ego
state to another. Box 5.1 illustrates the three ego states through
an extract from a fictional conversation at a party.

All three ego states have survival value for the individual and
the species. Each is appropriate in certain circumstances, so that
a person who habitually exhibits a single ego state will have a
noticeably limited social repertoire. For example, the person
whose ego state is predominantly Parent is likely to be kind and
nurturing, but may also be perceived as patronizing and lacking
in spontaneity. The habitual Adult will be very concerned with
practicalities of the present reality, but may show little interest
in creative or intuitive ideas. The habitual Child, on the other
hand, is typically creative and fun-loving, but may also appear
shallow and amoral. An effective, well-rounded personality may
be defined as one in which an ego state appropriate to the social
situation is always displayed, and in which the behaviour patterns of each are coherent with one another.

Ego states and illness behaviour

The operations of the Parent, Adult and Child in day-to-day social life can be illustrated by the decision to seek medical attention when ill. Figuratively, the Parent might say 'You should see the doctor when sick'. This would represent an attitude and behaviour learned from a real parent earlier in life. The Adult might say 'I am concerned about the implications of my illness, and wonder if the doctor might be able to help'. The Child might say 'I know the doctor will look after me'. In this example, the three 'voices' are consistent. In other circumstances they may not be. From the transactional perspective, the patient who starts a consultation by saying to the doctor 'I don't know if you can help with this, but I thought I ought to see you about it' is communicating that her Parent has decided that she should consult, but her Adult is not convinced of the value of doing so. The doctor could respond to the patient's Parent ('I am very glad you came to see me') or to her Adult ('Tell me how you think I might be able to help').

Analysing interactions

Transactional analysis gains its name from Berne's use of the word 'transaction' to refer to the combination of a single stimulus and a single response as a unit of social action. Thus, a conversation between two people consists of a chain of transactions, each spoken response becoming, in turn, the stimulus of the next transaction. Three types of transaction are distinguished: complementary, crossed and ulterior.

In a *complementary* transaction, the ego state that is addressed is the one that responds. The third and sixth transactions in Box 5.1 are complementary. During a consultation, the patient's Adult may converse with the doctor's Adult, or the patient's Child may interact with the doctor's Parent. In both cases, the series of transactions would be complementary and, irrespective of whether the Child–Parent interaction is appropriate to the professional relationship, would probably continue with no sense of discomfort on either side.

In a *crossed* transaction, the ego state that is addressed is not the one that responds. The first and second transactions in Box 5.1 provide examples. Another example was seen in the transference reaction described in Chapter 4, in which attempts by the doctor's Adult to speak to the patient's Adult were answered by the patient's Child speaking to the doctor's Parent (see Box 4.1).

An *ulterior* transaction is one in which two different messages are communicated simultaneously. The *social-level* exchange is typically indicated by the verbal content, and is usually Adult–Adult or Parent–Parent. The *psychological-level* communication is typically non-verbal, and is often Child–Child or Child–Parent. Ulterior transactions can often be observed at the start of a party, as couples indicate an inclination or disinclination to increase their level of intimacy while conversing about an emotionally neutral topic. The social-level transaction is usually Adult–Adult and the psychological transaction Child–Child. For example:

Lesley: How long have you known Mike? (Adult's verbal communication)
(Will you play with me later?) (Child's non-verbal message)
Kerry: About a year now. (Adult)
(Yes please!) (Child)

Berne has pointed out that the behavioural outcome of an ulterior transaction typically reflects the message at the psychological level rather than that at the social level, and such outcomes may be observed later at the same party.

The doctor may become aware of double messages in the consulting room. For example, the patient who says 'I'd like some more of those tablets, doctor' while acting in a vaguely threatening manner is communicating verbally with the doctor's Adult. At the same time, the patient's Parent is seeking to intimidate the doctor's Child. More subtle is the request 'I know you don't like prescribing appetite suppressants, doctor, but my old GP used to give them to me and they helped me such a lot'. Here the social-level communication is again directed to the doctor's Adult, but there is also an implicit appeal from the patient's Child to the doctor's nurturing Parent.

It is important to be aware of the power of psychological-level transactions, and of the way in which they may be masked by the parallel social-level exchange. Often the clue to a double communication from the patient is a momentary sense of confusion, or uncertainty about how to respond. Reflection may reveal that the patient is communicating one message to the doctor's Adult or Parent, and another to his Parent or Child. How the doctor responds can then be a matter of conscious choice. Options include responding only to the social-level communication, challenging the psychological-level message, or exploring the issues further. To use the example from the previous paragraph:

Patient: I know you don't like prescribing appetite suppressants, doctor, but my old GP used to give them to me and they helped me such a lot.

Doctor: You're quite right. I don't prescribe them, I'm afraid. (Social-level response)

Or: I'd like to help you, but I don't feel comfortable prescribing something because that is what another doctor used to do. (Challenging the psychological-level message)

Or: Perhaps you could tell me more about the reasons why you feel you need them? (Exploring the issues)

Of course, doctors are also capable of transmitting double messages to patients. Such communications are of their nature dishonest, even though the doctor may be unconscious of the psychological-level component. They may also be threatening, confusing or downright harmful to the patient. The key to prevention is to pay attention to any strong feelings that develop towards the patient, and to avoid communicating these within the consultation. An exception might be an explicit statement, made with clear therapeutic intent. For example, 'I'm very worried about you, and I think you should come and see me more regularly about your diabetes'.

Finally, it is of interest that much successful advertising of pharmaceutical products makes use of ulterior transactions; see Box 5.2 for examples.

Box 5.2 **Ulterior communications in pharmaceutical marketing**

Ferner and Scott (1994) surveyed advertisements for pharmaceutical products in medical journals, and identified five kinds of dishonest and mixed messages. Although the two authors did not use the theory of transactional analysis to interpret their observations, such an analysis is illuminating and suggests that ulterior communications are common in pharmaceutical advertising.

The five advertising techniques identified by Ferner and Scott were as follows:

- *Showing doctors as they might wish themselves to be.* For example, one advertisement showed a woman's confident face. She looked intelligent, mature yet handsome, kindly but determined. The accompanying text read: 'She's a GP. She relies on [antibiotic] for her vulnerable bronchitics. Made for you. By [drug company].' The message that one particular doctor favours a particular antibiotic for the treatment of bronchitis is hardly news, but is accompanied by a psychological-level message to the reader's nurturing Parent.
- *Adding to the reader's worries.* An advertisement for an H2 antagonist, before the era of widespread *Helicobacter pylori* eradication therapy, showed a volcano at first quiescent and then in fiery eruption. The accompanying text encouraged long-term maintenance treatment with a warning directed at the reader's fearful Child to 'consider an ulcer extinct at your patient's peril'.
- *Inviting the reader to participate in a puzzle.* A series of advertisements for a different H2 antagonist hid the initial letter of the product's brand name within pictures of rugged landscapes, perhaps inviting the reader's Child out to play.
- *Advertising by contagion.* Pictures in drug advertisements often imply attributes of the product that cannot be claimed in the text. An advertisement for a diuretic was accompanied by a photograph of a hand turning the tap of a burette containing urine; a message to the reader's Parent, perhaps, that he or she can exert precise control

over the patient's body. Another advertisement, for a hypnotic, was accompanied by a picture of a child asleep with a cuddly teddy bear. This image seems calculated to appeal to the reader's nurturing Parent.

- *Offering the reader a limited set of choices.* An advertisement for an antidepressant showed an array of stylized faces. Forty-one were miserable and coloured blue, the forty-second was cheerful and coloured yellow. This had been achieved through exercising 'the simple choice' of prescribing the antidepressant whose name was underlined in yellow and juxtaposed with a stylized yellow sun. The implied choice ignores other antidepressants, and non-drug treatments. This was the only advertising technique identified by Ferner and Scott that did not employ an ulterior communication for its intended behavioural effect. Instead, a restricted version of reality is offered to the reader's Adult.

Playing games in the consultation

One of the most useful ideas to emerge from the theory of transactional analysis is that of game playing. Games in this context are not light-hearted, trivial activities; a few are played to the death. A *game* is a series of transactions that adheres to the formula

$$C + G = R \rightarrow S \rightarrow X \rightarrow P$$

(Berne 1972). This can be read as 'con plus gimmick equals response, leading to switch, leading to crossup, ending in payoff.' The initiator starts by issuing a *con*; this is an ulterior invitation to the other person to join in the game. If the second person accepts the invitation, this is because they have a *gimmick*, defined as a weakness or need that leads them to respond to the con. Indeed, they may have invited the initiator to issue the con by exposing their gimmick. Following the second player's *response* to the con, the initiator shifts ground, making the *switch*. The second player is likely to feel a moment of confusion at the resulting *crossup*. The final outcome is a *payoff* of some kind of psychological gain for the initiator, and bad feelings for the second player. For example:

Patient: Do you think I will get better, doctor? (Con)
Doctor: Of course you will. (Response)
Patient: That's what you told my neighbour, but look how bad she is now. (Switch)

Berne called this game 'Whammy'. It will be familiar to many doctors, and highlights the dangers of providing unthinking reassurance. In transactional terms, the patient's initial utterance on the social level is a request for information from the doctor's Adult. Psychologically, she is seeking reassurance from his omniscient Parent. The doctor's Parent provides this, perhaps against the better judgement of his Adult. The patient's switch is again an ulterior communication, directed to the doctor's Adult at a social level, but to his Parent psychologically. The patient's payoff is in putting the doctor in his place: he is not all-knowing, and the patient is wiser than he about some things. A more useful response from the doctor might have been to enquire what, in particular, the patient was worried about.

Doctors initiate games as well, of course. One favourite is 'I'm only trying to help':

Doctor: You tell me that your neighbourhood has deteriorated over the last few years, and now you are afraid to leave the house at night. Why don't you move?
Patient: Well, I like my house, doctor, and all my friends live in the area.
Doctor: I was just trying to help.

The motivation for the doctor to play this game is that he can pretend to himself that he really is trying to help the patient, while failing to engage in any real sense with the patient's problem.

'I'm only trying to help' interlocks beautifully with the game of 'Why don't you . . . Yes but'. Skilled players can spin this combination out for years. Another interlocking game is 'See what you made me do':

Doctor: We know you have a weak back, and it is made worse by all the lifting you have to do at work. I think you should ask your boss for a lighter job.
Patient: That's a good idea, doctor.
Doctor (some weeks later): Did you speak with your boss?
Patient: Yes, he gave me the sack.

These examples highlight the dangers of offering advice to patients on how they should live their lives, something that doctors often feel that they should do. The solution is not to avoid addressing psychosocial problems and issues of lifestyle, but to approach them differently and in a collaborative manner with the patient. This point is taken up further in Chapter 8.

Recognizing and responding to a game

We learn to play games as children, and continue because we get psychological gains that offset the negative aspects of the payoff. Typically, we do not recognize games in which we are players, and Berne's formula can be a help in detecting and analysing our involvement. Freeling and Harris (1984) have listed a number of possible ways the doctor can respond if he perceives that he is being invited to play. These include the following:

• Play on regardless, because his need for the payoff exceeds his sense of professional responsibility.
• Play on unwillingly because he has no other options; at least he will know why he is going to lose!
• Play deliberately and knowingly, out of compassion or with the intention of subsequently discussing the dynamic of the game with the patient (not a little skill is required to do this successfully).
• Decline the invitation, without explanation. A vigorous reaction may be expected from the patient, which the patient–doctor relationship may not survive.
• Respond in a way that prevents the switch, as in the discussion of 'Whammy' above; this is often the most appropriate approach, and may be illustrated with another example, this time of 'Wooden leg':

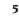

Patient: My chest is much better now, doctor. (Con)
Doctor: That's great. I think you should be back at work in the next week or so. (Response)
Patient: I really want to, but I don't know. My knee is still bad. (Switch)

'Wooden leg' is short for 'What do you expect from a man with a wooden leg?'. The patient's reason for not returning to work may be entirely valid, in which case he is not game playing. However, it is quite possible that a bad knee is not of itself sufficient reason for staying off work, although that would certainly depend on the nature of the patient's occupational skills, and the employment opportunities that are available to him.

'Wooden leg' is played when a disability can be offered as a plausible reason to be excused from social and personal obligations, and gives further insight into the mechanism of secondary gain described in the previous chapter. It allows the player to be free of blame and to get sympathy from casual acquaintances, and it provides a way of avoiding a more honest self-appraisal. Furthermore, the switch makes it difficult for the doctor to continue with the topic of the patient's return to work; after all, he forgot to enquire after the state of the patient's knee, and it would be churlish of him to pursue the matter further at this stage. As in 'Why don't you . . . Yes but' and 'See what you made me do' the doctor's gimmick was revealed when he suggested to the patient how he should live his life. The doctor could have avoided the crossup and payoff by asking 'Have you given any thought to going back to work?'. This would not prevent the patient from playing 'Wooden leg' with other people and with himself, but would give the doctor more room to negotiate following the patient's reply.

The development of transactional analysis

Eric Berne continued developing his theory up to the time of his death in 1970. *What Do You Say after You Say Hello?*, published posthumously (Berne 1972), outlines the theory as he understood it towards the end of his life. It discusses in particular the development of life scripts, which are important in psychotherapy based on transactional analysis (Stewart 1989), and which provide further insights into the motivations for game playing. The game formula outlined in the previous section is taken from *What Do You Say after You Say Hello?* and differs significantly from that described in Berne's earlier book, *Games People Play* (Berne 1964). Many of the 'games' in the earlier book lack a switch, and consist of a sequence of ulterior transactions for which many modern writers on transactional analysis would use the term 'racketeering' (Stewart 1992). Ulterior transactions of this form were discussed in the first section of this chapter.

In spite of claims by its apologists, the theory of transactional analysis is more descriptive than explanatory of human behaviour. Nevertheless, the theory does provide a colourful language for describing the processes of social interaction, and a number of useful models for interpreting those descriptions. It can also offer clues to the likely outcomes of different behaviours in social settings, and can provide a valuable guide to action within the consultation.

6 Discourse in the consultation

A people are as healthy and confident as the stories they tell themselves.... Only those who have lived, suffered, thought deeply, loved profoundly, known joy and the tragic penumbra of things tell truly wonderful stories.

(Ben Okri 1996: 18, 23)

In a famous study that was undertaken in a medical out-patient clinic, but is relevant to clinical practice in other settings, the physician wrote down a provisional diagnosis for each consecutive new patient after reading the family doctor's referral letter, again after taking a history, and again after examining the patient. These provisional diagnoses were compared with the accepted final diagnosis, two months later. A provisional diagnosis that agreed with the final diagnosis was made after reading the referral letter and taking the history in 66 out of 80 patients. The diagnosis was changed for only six patients after physical examination, and for only seven following laboratory investigations. The researchers concluded that in their particular setting 'the diagnosis can be made and the management of the patient can be accurately forecast on the basis of the history in three-quarters of the new patients seen' (Hampton *et al.* 1975: 489).

This conclusion ignored the contribution from information in the referral letter, but was nevertheless consistent with other research on the diagnostic process which suggests that experienced doctors reach the majority of their diagnostic hypotheses on the basis of the history, and then use the examination and investigations to distinguish between the possibilities that they have identified, and to screen for other rare but significant conditions (Gale and Marsden 1983; Kassirer 1989).

In general practice, the conversation between patient and doctor is arguably even more significant for diagnosis and assessment than it is in the medical out-patient clinic. Indeed, many consultations are successfully completed without any examination being undertaken or investigations arranged. Furthermore, the provision of information, negotiation of an agreed management plan, and many other tasks, are necessarily dependent on verbal interaction. Clearly, the talking that goes on in the consultation is of considerable practical importance, and has been the subject of a substantial number of research studies, undertaken from a range of theoretical perspectives. In this chapter I will review several of these perspectives, which between them offer a number of practical lessons for the consultation in family practice.

Diagnostic and prescriptive styles

Doctors Talking to Patients was the title of one of the first systematic studies of conversations in general practice (Byrne and Long 1976). Although the research was undertaken during the early 1970s, many of the observations remain pertinent today. Over 2500 consultations were recorded on audio-tape, and subsequently analysed. The researchers categorized the doctors' verbal behaviour into four diagnostic styles, and seven prescriptive styles. The diagnostic styles were labelled as follows:

* gathering information;
* analysing and probing;
* clarifying and interpreting;
* listening and reflecting.

This range of diagnostic styles was well illustrated by the different responses to a patient's utterance such as 'Well, I'm feeling run down. I've got a pain in my back, and I just feel tired all day'. Replies that the investigators recorded included the following:

* 'Tell me. Just where is this pain?' (gathering information).
* 'Do you have headaches and pains behind the eyes?' (analysing and probing).

- 'What do you mean by "I feel tired all day"? (clarifying and interpreting).
- 'Yes, go on' (listening and reflecting).

The 'prescriptive styles' described how the doctor approached the development of a management plan. Byrne and Long identified the following:

- Doctor instructs the patient.
- Doctor makes his decision and tells the patient what it is.
- Doctor sells his decision to the patient.
- Doctor presents a tentative decision, subject to change.
- Doctor presents the problem, seeks suggestions and makes decisions.
- Doctor defines the limits and asks the patient to make a decision.
- Doctor permits the patient to make her own decision.

It can be seen that each set of styles constitutes a spectrum. At one extreme, the doctor's utterances reflect his medical knowledge, with little use made of the experience and knowledge of the patient. At the other extreme, the doctor facilitates verbalization of the patient's ideas and adds little of his own understanding. The researchers observed that most doctors stayed with a limited range of only one or two adjacent diagnostic styles, and two or three prescriptive styles. Both they, and the study participants, argued that for maximal effectiveness the doctor should match his style to the patient, the problem and the context. Other writers have made a similar suggestion (Smith and Hoppe 1991). However, the study by Byrne and Long, and subsequent research (Roter *et al.* 1997), suggest that few doctors vary their style in this way.

Asymmetrical conversations

Byrne and Long's observation, that doctors were able to maintain their preferred style in consultations with a wide range of patients about a great variety of problems, illustrates the asymmetry of power that exists in the patient–doctor relationship.

Verbal interactions between patients and doctors are typically asymmetrical in other ways, too. There is of course an asymmetry of topic, as it is the patient's health that is under consideration, not that of the doctor. There is also an asymmetry of tasks between the patient and doctor, and hence an asymmetry in the nature and interplay of their utterances.

This latter asymmetry has been studied using an approach to the analysis of verbal interactions called *conversation analysis* (Frankel 1989; Psathas 1995). The focus of conversation analysis is on the sequential structure of the interaction, and on the ways in which the participants achieve this. The content and structure of each utterance are examined in detail, as is its relationship to the utterances that precede and follow. Of particular interest is the work of ten Have (1991). He showed how doctors tend to monopolize the initiative in the consultation, so that each new topic of discussion is introduced by the doctor. For example:

Doctor: Does the pain wake you at night?
Patient: No.
Doctor: Have you ever vomited up blood?

Here the doctor has, presumably, made a mental note of the patient's reply to his first question, but has then gone on to ask about another issue in his next utterance. Sometimes doctors do respond to the patient, but often in a non-committal way:

Doctor: Have you vomited at all, in the last few days?
Patient: No.
Doctor: Mmm . . . and the diarrhoea, have you noticed any blood in it?

As ten Have has pointed out, doctors tend not to justify their questions, or to give much indication of what they think about the answers, at least while they are continuing to seek further information. By doing this, they ensure that the conversation stays focused on the experiences, ideas and feelings of the patient.

Patients may ask questions themselves, but rarely do so early in the consultation while the doctor is himself seeking information. If they do, then the doctor is likely to regain the initiative within the same utterance as his answer:

Patient: What do you think caused it, doctor?
Doctor: I don't know yet. I need to ask you some more questions. Have you ever had a problem like this before?

A major contribution of conversation analysis has been to provide a deeper understanding of the ways in which power is both displayed and maintained in the patient–doctor interaction. By tending to monopolize the initiative in asking questions, at least while seeking information, and by withholding information about his own thoughts and emotional responses, the doctor displays the privilege associated with his role. At the same time, by behaving in these ways, the doctor ensures that it is information about the patient, and not the doctor, that is disclosed during the interaction. Thus, asymmetry of enquiry and disclosure both reflect and help to maintain the power relationship.

The hermeneutic circle

Doctors are taught to listen to the patient's story of her illness, to extract key elements, and to construct a history from these. A recent consultation of mine started as follows:

Doctor: How can I help?
Patient: I've been pretty sick, Doc. I keep coughing up blood.
Doctor: That must be scary. When did this start?
Patient: About three days ago.

In the technical language of medicine, this patient presented with a three-day history of haemoptysis. The elements that doctors are taught to extract in this way are mainly those with diagnostic or prognostic value in the current medical explanatory model. Little (1995: 155) has suggested that:

When clinicians 'take' a medical history [they] turn the patient's narrative to text, removing the discourse from the patient's lived experience. Doctors assume a set of editorial functions, determined by their need to observe linguistic conventions that may be entirely alien to the patient.

In fact, doctors do more than this. Through their questions and other utterances, they coach the patient to produce the kind of narrative that they want. M. Balint (1973) described how doctors may use selective attention and selective neglect towards the various elements of the patient's story in order to do this (see Chapter 4). Presumably, the more biomedically minded doctor will tend to ignore the psychosocial aspects of the patient's account, and to enquire most deeply into her physical symptoms. Conversely, the doctor who aims at whole-person care will maintain a broader focus. However, even the latter doctor may be inclined to view the patient's narrative, once spoken, as text that is open to objective analysis. That is, although different doctors may elicit a story that differs in content and emphasis, the interpretation of the elicited story becomes a simple matter of clinical method – that of recognizing typical symptom complexes, for example.

This is the traditional position of hermeneutics, the study of textual analysis. The *hermeneutic circle* describes the process of developing an understanding of a text by examining the meaning of each section of it, and relating these sections to each other and to the text as whole. Thus, the analysis moves from the whole text to its parts, and back to the whole. Traditionally, the reader approaches the text without preconceptions, open-mindedly and without prejudice. More recently, it has been argued that this is not possible. Not only do we approach *all* texts, including patients' narratives, with prejudices borne of previous experiences, but it is these very prejudices and preconceptions that make understanding possible (Outhwaite 1985).

Taking as an example the fragment of narrative reported at the start of this section, the somewhat parsimonious interpretation that the patient had a three-day history of haemoptysis does not do full justice to the richness of meaning in her utterances. In particular, the expression 'I've been pretty sick' suggests that there was more to her illness than the fact of having been coughing up blood. In addition, it was not difficult to make the empathic assumption that coughing up blood is a frightening experience. A richer interpretation of the patient's opening utterances might be that she presented with a three-day history of haemoptysis, which was likely to have been a frightening experience for her, and that she might also have been feeling ill in other ways. (I must confess to the benefit of hindsight here; the patient did have a number of other symptoms.)

It seems that when a doctor 'takes a history', he brings to the interaction a range of preconceptions that are borne of previous experience, and that influence both how he reacts to the patient's narrative, and how he interprets it. Indeed, the very story that the patient produces will reflect in part the doctor's interpretations and consequent responses. The danger is not that the doctor influences the patient's narrative – that is unavoidable – but that he does so without understanding. Doctors need to reflect continually on their values and prejudices, and to be aware of how these impact directly on their clinical encounters.

Telling and hearing stories

The consultation can be seen as a context in which both patient and doctor spend much of their time telling each other stories. I find this quite a fruitful perspective, especially as we tell and hear stories in a wide variety of situations, and the lessons learned are often transferable. Most patients attend the doctor with a story to tell, one that they may well have discussed with friends and relatives (see Chapter 1) and may have sat rehearsing in the waiting room. Implicit or explicit in this story is the patient's reason for attending the doctor; not necessarily what is wrong physically, but the tasks that the patient wants the doctor to perform (Launer 1995). Yet many doctors interrupt the patient before she has finished speaking. Not only is this poor manners, but the doctor gives up his best chance of discovering what it is that the patient is most concerned about, and what it is that she actually wants from the consultation.

The patient's opening statement

Doctors sometimes argue that if they do not interrupt the patient's story early on, and seek diagnostically specific details in the history, the patient may waste considerable time talking about issues of no diagnostic relevance. Interestingly, in a study of 74 consultations in a primary care clinic, Beckman and Frankel

(1984) found that if the doctor did not interrupt then most patients finished talking within 50 seconds, and none took longer than 150 seconds. In another study, Linfors and Neelon (1981) arranged for 55 unselected ambulatory care patients, attending for comprehensive medical assessment, to be first interviewed using non-directive techniques and then reinterviewed using a structured questionnaire. Of the 269 clinically important problems that were identified, 198 (74 per cent) were elicited by the initial interview, and a further 71 (26 per cent) by questionnaire. Few of the latter were subsequently acted upon, however. The investigators concluded that 'an open-ended interview, undertaken with the intention of identifying all the patient's health problems, detects those problems well' (Linfors and Neelon 1981: 426). Other research has shown benefit from including systematic questions to screen for health promotion opportunities (Ramsey *et al.* 1998). However, these can be left to the end of the interview, and the evidence suggests that time is well spent listening without interruption to the patient's initial account of her symptoms.

The technique of such listening is worth examining. Often it is possible to sit and attend to the patient's story without saying anything. However, in the study referred to above, Beckman and Frankel (1984) demonstrated that if the doctor uttered *continuers* such as 'mmh hmh', 'go on' and 'I see' at appropriate moments then the patient was likely to introduce new topics and concerns into her narrative. In contrast, questions by the doctor that referred to a particular topic in the patient's story were highly effective at interrupting the narrative, and it was unlikely that the patient would subsequently return to an open-ended account of her story. An example of such an interruption by the doctor is given below:

Patient: Well, doctor, when I woke up this morning, I had this sharp pain in the side of my chest.
Doctor: Is the pain worse when you breathe in?

Significantly, utterances by the doctor that are frequently described as facilitators of open-ended interviewing, such as *elaborators*, *recompleters* and *statements*, also acted as highly effective interruptors during the patient's opening statement:

Patient: Last night, I woke with a terrible pain in my belly, and it was ages before I got back to sleep.
Doctor: Tell me more about the pain. (Elaborator)
Or: Ages before you got back to sleep. (Recompleter)
Or: You woke last night with a terrible pain in your belly. (Statement).

Beckman and Frankel observed that patients rarely introduced new topics following such interjections by the doctor. While elaborators, recompleters and statements have a clear place in eliciting further details of the patient's story after the opening statement, their use during it focuses attention on particular issues and may inhibit subsequent disclosure of the full range of the patient's concerns.

Once again, further research is needed in this area, but on the available evidence doctors should listen without interruption to the whole of the patient's opening statement, uttering only continuers if interjections are judged useful. At the end of the statement, the doctor might invite further issues by summarizing what the patient has just said, or perhaps with a broad open question such as 'Is there anything else?'. The concerns raised by the patient can then be explored in greater depth.

The patient's metaphors and the two agendas

A familiar device in storytelling is the use of *metaphor*. Metaphors have the intent of conveying a similarity in the attributes of two otherwise dissimilar things. For example:

You are the bows from which your children as living arrows are sent forth.
The archer sees the mark upon the path of the infinite, and He bends you with His might that His arrows may go swift and far.
Let your bending in the Archer's hand be for gladness;
For even as He loves the arrow that flies, so He loves also the bow that is stable.

(Gibran 1976: 20, 23)

Patients' metaphors may point to additional layers of meaning that are not apparent from the primary narrative. For example, the patient who says 'I feel so trapped by my disease' may be communicating something about the functional impact of her illness that the doctor needs to hear and consider (Shapiro 1993). This example demonstrates the value of listening for words and phrases that may not be of much diagnostic or biological relevance, but may be of considerable personal meaning for the patient. Platt (1995) has suggested that failure by doctors to listen out for such statements, to acknowledge them and to explore the meaning behind them, is a potent cause of misunderstanding between doctor and patient. He gives the example of a brief dialogue that will be familiar to all clinicians:

> *Doctor:* How long have you had the chest pain?
> *Patient:* Since I moved to Denver.
> *Doctor:* And how long ago was that?
> *Patient:* About three years.

Clearly, the duration of the pain is likely to be of great diagnostic significance, but the doctor has missed the opportunity to ask about its connection in the patient's mind with her move to Denver.

Levenstein *et al.* (1986) have elaborated the notion of *two agendas*. The patient's agenda reflects her ideas and questions about her illness, her hopes and expectations of the doctor, her feelings, her fears and her problems of living. The doctor's agenda is concerned with correct diagnosis of the patient's complaints. It is the doctor's responsibility to respect the patient's agenda and to reconcile this with his own (Smith and Hoppe 1991). This entails acknowledging and responding to affective cues (see Chapter 3); exploring the meaning behind statements that seem important to the patient, even if their relevance is not obvious to the doctor; using open questions and facilitation when asking about symptoms; seeking the patient's views, fears, questions, hopes and expectations; and summarizing as a way of integrating the two agendas into a single narrative (Brown *et al.* 1986).

Healing stories

Telling stories provides a way of ordering experience. As we describe an experience to others, we define it, locate it in relation to ourselves, interpret it and evaluate it. The experience of sickness can have a profound impact on our lives, but much of that impact is mediated via the stories that we tell ourselves. If this is the case, then as doctors we have both an opportunity and a responsibility to help our patients tell illness stories that empower rather than disempower (Greenhalgh and Hurwitz 1999).

There seem to be two aspects to such therapeutic listening. The first is what Kleinman (1988) has described as *empathic witnessing*. This means listening to the patient's story with a commitment to understanding how it must feel to be that person, living that person's life and experiencing that person's illness. Shapiro (1993) has argued that in order to listen in this way, the doctor should bear in mind the fundamentals of textual criticism. He needs to become intimate with the text of the story; he must be willing to immerse himself within the world created by this text; he must respect the text and not do intentional violence to its meanings; and he must be committed to exploring and understanding these meanings. Weingarten and Worthen (1997), in an entirely unsentimental account of their own experiences of serious illness, emphasize their need to have their illness texts heard in ways that elaborate but do not challenge the basic integrity of their stories.

The second aspect of therapeutic listening can be described as the co-creation, by patient and doctor, of stories that heal rather than harm (Brody 1994). When listening, the doctor has a responsibility to question, to challenge and to facilitate the patient in exploring the assumptions and meanings behind her own story. To give an example, the patient who says that she cannot stop smoking, that she has tried before, and that she has always started again, has become trapped in a harmful story. The doctor can help her explore possible alternative stories by asking questions such as 'Tell me about the last time you tried to stop. What else was going on in your life at that time? Are things different now? Why do you think you started smoking again? Is there anything you could do to change that?'

In conclusion, Launer (1995) has suggested that while doctors tend to see *actions* such as prescribing, surgery and referral as the principal means of relieving suffering, we also have a role as *witnesses* to our patients' distress, and as *facilitators* of the quest for new meanings in their stories.

7 | The family and chronic illness

Establishing a relationship where families feel they are with someone who is ready, unafraid and unembarrassed to understand what they face – be this fear of death, envy for the health of others, or irritation with comments about their courage – cannot be over-emphasised.

(Jenny Altschuler 1997: 62)

Our families provide the context within which we experience illness, in both ourselves and others. It is one of the defining characteristics of primary medical care that patients are assessed and managed within the context of their families; this context is ignored in many secondary care settings. Much of the research on family processes and their interactions with processes of illness has focused on biological families with mother, father, children and a network of relatives (Eiser 1990). However, family structures vary enormously, and a useful definition is 'a group of people, living together or in close contact, who take care of one another' (modified from Patterson 1995: 47).

In Chapter 1, I outlined the ways in which family and other social processes influence how we interpret and respond to illness. In this chapter, I will review some of the ways in which families may be affected by illness, especially if chronic or severe, and I will explore the implications for care by the family doctor. In the second part of the chapter I will outline the biopsychosocial model of illness, and discuss how this may help the doctor to organize her response. Emotional and relationship problems, which often involve family processes, will be discussed in Chapter 8.

Effects of illness on the family

The impact of illness falls not only on the individual with symptoms, but also on those who live with the sick person and attend to his needs. There are three key areas of family functioning that are typically affected by illness, especially if it is severe, prolonged or life-threatening. These areas are:

• relationships within the family;
• coping with practical tasks;
• relationships outside the family.

The effectiveness with which a family adapts to meet the challenges in each of these areas tends to reflect the resources that they had available before the illness became manifest (Eiser 1990). Resources may be psychological or practical. Psychological resources refer to the mental health of individual family members, and to the relationships that they have with each other and with the outside world. Practical resources relate to housing, transport, and especially income and savings.

The general practitioner has a responsibility to support the patient's family in coping with the changes that result from illness. This role is particularly important when the patient is a child, is severely disabled, exhibits behaviour that challenges the family in some way, or is terminally ill. In this section I will review the changes that may occur in each of the three areas listed above, and then discuss the implications for care in the consultation.

Relationships within the family

Confronted with sickness, each family member has to find a way of redefining their expectations of themselves, and their relationships with one another. The sick person may feel fear at his prognosis, may grieve for lost hopes and dreams, and may also feel embarrassment, anger, guilt or disgust at the manifestations of his illness. Other members of the family may have similar feelings, and may blame themselves, the sick person or others for what has happened. It is important for the family doctor to acknowledge expressions of such feelings empathically, but without colluding with them.

Illness is frequently seen as disempowering. It often is, but paradoxically may also increase the power that a sick person exercises within the family. He may use illness as an excuse for avoiding certain tasks, so that others have to undertake these roles. The sick person may be dependent on others to care for his physical needs, whether or not they wish to do so. The exercise of such power, wittingly or not, may be resented by other members of the family. One member of the family may form an *alliance* with the patient and so share in his power (Williams 1989). Often the person to do this is the main caregiver. Once again, it is important for the family doctor to avoid colluding with such an alliance; to do so can reinforce it, and may reduce the doctor's availability to other members of the family.

Relationships between members of the family other than the sick person may be affected, often adversely. There may be financial pressures to cope with, interrupted sleep, reduced opportunity for intimacy, and other stressors. When a child is sick, one or both parents may focus most of their energies on caring for him to the exclusion of his siblings and the other parent. In time, this may impact on the quality of the marital relationship, and will also mean that the parent has less time to devote to the developmental needs of the other children. Research has consistently shown that mothers of chronically sick children have poorer mental health than mothers of healthy children (Eiser 1990). The siblings of sick children may exhibit behavioural and other problems. The impact of illness on a family may not be all negative, however. Individual members may discover within themselves an increased capacity for compassion, sensitivity and understanding. In the family as a whole, communication and intimacy may be enhanced.

Coping with practical tasks

Many illnesses present the family with novel tasks and challenges. Some of these are related to the illness itself, such as supervising medication, providing physical care, and arranging clinic visits. Others reflect changes in the daily routine. Someone else may have to fetch the shopping, get the family up in the morning, or feed the cat. In addition, the family may experience a reduction in their income and other changes in their circumstances (Covinsky *et al.* 1994).

Coping with the practical challenges of illness requires flexibility, with family members communicating clearly and openly, respecting one other, and being willing to support and help one another (Gerson *et al.* 1993). Research has consistently shown that a positive perception of family and other social support is associated with a more favourable outcome in a wide range of diseases (Kriegsman *et al.* 1995; Penninx *et al.* 1996).

Relationships outside the family

It has been said that illness increases the permeability of the boundary between the family and its social environment (Altschuler 1997). Health professionals and others may adopt roles that were previously the exclusive domain of parents or siblings. New relationships must be forged, and existing ones redefined.

The social environment is often a source of encouragement and additional resources. Emotional support and practical help may come from neighbours, friends, relatives, members of the family's religious group, and others. Many seriously ill or disabled people would not be able to live at home without such assistance. However, help from outside the family, including care from health professionals, can have its disadvantages. Some helpers are concerned more with meeting their own needs for love and self-esteem than with addressing the needs of the sick person, and may disrupt emotional relationships within the family. Others may be quick to label the family as 'over-protective' or 'enmeshed'. The self-esteem of members of the family may be undermined by provision of unwanted support, or by such labels, and the family's capacity for coping may be compromised.

Sometimes, one member of a family becomes a *gatekeeper*, and acts as the main conduit of information between the family and others. This may meet emotional and practical needs, but problems can occur (see Box 7.1).

Box 7.1 An inappropriate gatekeeper

A Somali refugee living in England attended her general practitioner with her uncle and 12-year-old son. These three people were the only known survivors of their once large family. The woman spoke no English and the uncle very little. Her son understood and spoke both English and Somali. He acted as interpreter, and hence gatekeeper, for most transactions between the family and their new English-speaking environment.

The son explained to the doctor that his mother was sick and had abdominal discomfort. He could not say when these symptoms had started, and was not able to describe any other features of the illness. The doctor's specific questions did not elicit further details. Examination of the woman's abdomen did not demonstrate any abnormalities. The doctor asked for a urine specimen for analysis, and arranged for the woman to attend two days later when the practice interpreter would be present.

At the follow-up consultation, when neither son nor uncle was present, the doctor learned via the interpreter that the woman had suffered heavy, painful, frequent periods for several years, and that this was why she had sought medical attention. However, she had been embarrassed about explaining the details via her son. Families may be forced for very practical reasons to use one member as a gatekeeper, but the role may not always be appropriate for that person or for the family. Ultimately, it is the responsibility of the doctor, not the patient, to ensure that patient–doctor communication is clear and unambiguous.

Implications for care

How can the general practitioner assist patients and their families to cope with the demands and changes wrought by illness? Altschuler (1997) has emphasized the value to families of having a doctor who is willing to face these issues alongside them.

The quotation at the start of this chapter highlights the value of an ongoing relationship with a single doctor who accepts personal responsibility for the family's continuing care. Where it is impossible to provide such a commitment, then the doctor must at least ensure adequate follow-up by a colleague, and provide sufficient documentation in the medical record to enable this. Relationships with non-medical members of the practice team may also be significant in providing the family with ongoing support.

The doctor can only understand what the patient and family are facing if she is willing to *listen* to what they have to tell her. When asked what they value in a doctor, patients and relatives regularly indicate the importance of listening (Rees Lewis 1994; Buetow 1995). Other important tasks for the doctor include:

- managing the disease process, including intervening preventively, monitoring and referring;
- providing information, raising sensitive issues, and normalizing experiences;
- advocacy with other professionals;
- helping to prepare for the future;
- addressing narratives of blame.

Patients and their carers look to their doctors to provide them with information about their treatment, their prognosis and the resources that are available to them (see Box 7.2). In providing

---

Box 7.2   Resource needs of carers

Anderson (1987) summarized the findings of research into the needs of carers of people with chronic illness:

- information about disabilities and services;
- physical help;
- money;
- time for themselves;
- planned respite care;
- recognition of their work;
- continuity of support.

---

this information, the doctor may help to normalize their illness experience. Many patients and their families feel alienated by sickness, as if they are the only people to be touched by illness in an otherwise healthy world. This perception will be enhanced if they are avoided by members of their social network, which may be particularly likely in the case of mental illness or infectious disease. The knowledge that they are not alone, and that the doctor has met similar illnesses before, can be very helpful.

Often, patients and family members are embarrassed or otherwise reluctant to raise all the issues that concern them. The doctor may need to ask directly about such concerns, which often relate to sex or death. Patients who are recovering from myocardial infarction or gynaecological surgery, for example, may want to know when they can resume sexual activity. People with physical disabilities, particularly affecting the lower limbs, may require more detailed advice. Patients and families may also need help and support in preparing for what the future is likely to bring. When the illness is expected to lead to death, the doctor has a role in helping both patient and family to prepare for this through the provision of information, practical advice and emotional support (Parkes and Markus 1998).

Addressing narratives of blame

Reflecting and reinforcing emotions of anger, shame, anxiety and guilt, *narratives of blame* are common in families facing serious illness. The mother of a child with congenital heart disease may blame herself for some action during her pregnancy. The son of a woman with lung cancer may blame his father's cigarette smoking. Such narratives may or may not make sense in the light of current medical knowledge. Either way, they poison relationships, obstruct personal growth, and inhibit family members in supporting and helping one another. A useful approach to challenging such narratives has been outlined by Altschuler (1997):

- Acknowledge the sense of blame.
- Interrupt the blaming if possible, by exploring discrepancies with current medical knowledge.

- Explore the consequences of the blaming for relationships within the family.
- Highlight the failure of blaming to alter the illness and the suffering that it brings.
- Explore the emptiness and hurt behind the blaming.

It is important to remember that an unthinking remark by a health professional may be the original cause of much blaming, and to appreciate the power for both good and harm of what doctors say to patients.

Two principles and a warning

Two principles should underpin all contact with the families of ill patients. The first is that the doctor must be aware of the family's need to maintain a balance between the tasks associated with caring for their sick member, and the tasks associated with mutual growth and development. The second is that the doctor must at all times support, and not undermine, the work of members of the family. Doctors can come and go; members of the family may not have this choice. The dangers of colluding with expressions of blame, or with coalitions within the family, have been mentioned already, as have those of undertaking tasks that are the responsibility of family members. The example in Box 7.3 illustrates another potential pitfall.

Finally, the doctor must beware of projecting on to the patient's family beliefs, attitudes and assumptions that have their origin in her own family experience. No two families function in the same way, but the contrasts may be particularly apparent when patient and doctor hail from very different ethnic backgrounds. Most Western cultures, for example, emphasize the right (and even the responsibility) of the individual to make decisions about his or her medical care. Among other cultures, the family may be the locus of decision-making. The family existed before the patient arrived on the scene, and will continue to exist after he dies. The patient is part of the family, and it is the family who makes the decisions (Kleinman 1988).

Box 7.3   Disempowering the family

Both mother and father were present at a well child visit for Allison, a healthy, two-week-old baby girl. When the father asked how much formula Allison should be taking, the doctor calculated her requirement from the infant's weight, and answered the question. As he answered, the father looked triumphant, turned to Allison's mother and said 'You see, I *was* right'. The mother's eyes fell and her head slumped forward. Subsequently, she developed post-natal depression and required psychiatric treatment. The doctor who described this incident concluded: 'What I had interpreted as support and care for the baby turned out to have been a battle for the "better parent" role. The father had won, hands down' (Cohen 1995: 13).

With the advantage of hindsight it is easy to suggest that the doctor might more helpfully have responded to the father's question with one of his own: 'What is it that you are concerned about?' Requests for factual information are frequently straightforward and can be taken at face value. However, it is always worth wondering about the reasons for any question from a patient or family member, and perhaps exploring these before answering.

Family systems and the biopsychosocial model

Implicit in much of the discussion above is the notion of the family as a *system*. That is, a family consists of a number of elements that communicate to share information, and to interact in other ways. In the short term at least, the membership of a family tends to be fairly constant and the patterns of interaction, or *family dynamics*, tend to be relatively stable. Families are also *open* systems. Not only do family members interact with each other, they also interact with others outside the family system, including doctors and other health professionals, and these interactions may impact on the intra-family dynamics. Finally, families are part of a *hierarchy* of systems. They contain subsystems, such as those of parents and of siblings, and they are components of larger systems, such as churches or other community groups. It is this notion of a hierarchy that underpins the *biopsychosocial model* proposed by George Engel (1977; 1980).

The biopsychosocial model provides a useful organizing framework for understanding the processes that impact on health and illness from sub-cellular to political and societal levels. Engel proposed the model as an alternative to what he called the *biomedical model.* By the latter term Engel meant the application to medicine of the reductionist, analytic approach that is characteristic of much Western science. The biomedical model has served us well in elucidating the causes and pathological effects of disease. However, as Engel pointed out, this approach does not focus on the unit of medical care, the sick person, but on his component parts. The biopsychosocial model is intended to incorporate and extend the biomedical model to include the sick person, his family and his social environment. It is based on the notion of a hierarchy of systems ranging from sub-atomic particles, through atoms, molecules, organelles, cells, tissues, organs and organ systems to the individual person, and then through two-person dyads, the family, community, society and nation to the biosphere.

Systems can be identified at each level of this hierarchy as organized, dynamic wholes with a degree of stability of structure and function. The characteristics of the systems are qualitatively different at each level, so that different technologies are required for their investigation, different theories are needed for their understanding and different interventions are required to effect change. The systems at the different levels of the hierarchy are not, however, independent. Each system provides the environment for those lower in the hierarchy, and is a component of systems higher up. Thus, changes at one level may alter the structure and function of systems at other levels.

The value of Engel's biopsychosocial model is as an organizing framework for theories of disease at levels ranging from the sub-cellular to the socioeconomic. It suggests in general terms the potential for changes at one level to influence processes at another. In addition, the model can act as a reminder for the clinician to consider health-promoting interventions at multiple levels (see Box 7.4 for an example).

Box 7.4   A case of diabetic ulcers

A 62-year-old man, resident for many years in a Salvation Army hostel, has ulcers on his feet secondary to non-insulin dependent diabetes mellitus. Following assessment, appropriate interventions might include the following:

- hypoglycaemic medication (primary impact at cellular level);
- dietary advice (tissues and organs);
- referral to a chiropodist (tissues and organs);
- elucidation and discussion of relevant health beliefs and related fears and expectations of care (person);
- arrangements for follow-up and regular review (patient–practice system);
- negotiation with hostel for appropriate diet and care (family);
- lobbying for adequate community chiropody and dietetic services (community);
- voting and other political action in support of equity of access to health care (nation).

The biopsychosocial model has had a significant influence on research and clinical practice, particularly in North America. It has, however, been criticized on both theoretical and practical grounds (Launer and Lindsey 1997). The theoretical criticism reflects the constructionist nature of the model; systems are constructs in the mind of the beholder. While it is often useful to discuss systems, subsystems and their attributes as if they have independent existence, as with all theoretical constructs, there is the risk of confusing the map with the territory.

A practical problem is that the model is far too complex and all-encompassing to be applied routinely in every consultation in a busy medical practice. Herman (1989) has argued that the biomedical model is quite adequate much of the time, and that on occasion attempts to assess the psychosocial aspects of a patient's problem may distract the doctor from treating significant physical disease. On other occasions, the primary focus should be on psychosocial issues. Full biopsychosocial assessment and intervention may be appropriate in only a minority of consultations.

8 Emotional and psychosocial problems

> *The doctor in general practice has to learn to live with his patients in a much more unchanging world than often both would wish.*
>
> (Andrew Elder 1987: 54)

A core theme of this book has been the proposition that family doctors have a responsibility which extends beyond the prevention and treatment of physical disease to include emotional and psychosocial issues. Indeed, it is difficult to see how adequate care of physical illness could be offered without proper attention to psychological and social factors.

Patients are often apprehensive and worried when they consult the doctor, and many have levels of psychological distress that reach criteria for a formal diagnosis of depressive illness or anxiety disorder (Ustun and Sartorius 1995). Associated with such distress may be relationship difficulties, sexual assault, domestic violence, life crises, alcohol and drug misuse, or other problems. A few patients exhibit evidence of emotional distress, or describe significant psychosocial concerns, at the start of the consultation; others present with somatic symptoms or in other ways.

There are limitations in applying categorical classifications of mental illness, such as the *Diagnostic and Statistical Manual* (DSM) of the American Psychiatric Association, or the World Health Organization *International Classification of Disease* (ICD), to the range and variety of human misery seen in primary care. I will start this chapter by describing an alternative model for understanding psychological distress that provides a useful conceptual basis for guiding management in the community context. I will then discuss some of the implications for care in the consultation. In the next chapter, I will outline a number of approaches to understanding why many patients with emotional and psychosocial difficulties present initially with somatic symptoms, and discuss ways of responding helpfully to such presentations.

The biosocial model

The notion of *psychological distress* is a useful one in the community context, encompassing grief, anxiety and clinical depression, but extending beyond those constructs to include all states in which unpleasant emotions are associated with significant distress or disability. In their book *Common Mental Disorders*, Goldberg and Huxley (1992) reviewed research into the causes, manifestations and outcomes of psychological distress. They concluded that:

> Instead of the myriad of sub-divisions of minor illness to be found in the ICD or the DSM-III classifications . . . there are only a very limited number of ways that the human frame responds to psychological stress, and these are defined by two underlying dimensions of symptomatology: anxious symptoms on the one hand, and depressive symptoms on the other. These two dimensions are themselves correlated, and combinations of the two sets of symptoms are more common than either set on its own. The apparent diversity of common illnesses is because there are a number of ways of responding to the experience of symptoms of anxiety or depression, and each of these ways is associated with a cluster of highly characteristic symptoms which have attracted the various categories contained in official taxonomies.
>
> (Goldberg and Huxley 1992: 139)

Earlier in their book, Goldberg and Huxley proposed that we are all more or less vulnerable to psychological destabilization, depending on the nature and intensity of the various stressors that we meet in our lives. If we become destabilized, and hence emotionally distressed, the nature of the symptoms that we experience reflects an interaction between our individual predisposition and the stressors to which we are subject. Whether we

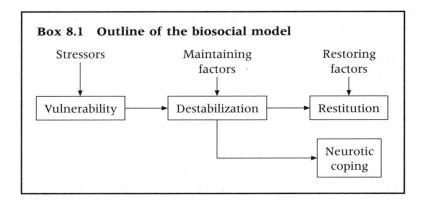

Box 8.1 Outline of the biosocial model

remain distressed, return to psychological stability, or develop neurotic coping mechanisms, depends on a range of maintaining and restoring factors, including the nature and quality of any health care that we receive. This model built on earlier work by Brown and Harris (1978; Brown 1987) and is outlined schematically in Box 8.1.

Vulnerability factors

Clearly, people vary in their susceptibility to psychological de-stabilization and emotional distress. Four groups of factors seem to be important in determining our individual vulnerability:

- childhood experiences;
- constitutional factors;
- current relationships;
- socioeconomic adversity.

Much research has been undertaken into the influence of *childhood experiences* on adult mental health. Although the findings of different studies are not altogether consistent with one another (Kagan and Zentner 1996) the available evidence suggests that maltreatment, sexual abuse, care by a depressed mother, parental disharmony, and possibly the loss of a parent, may all increase the risk of mental illness in adult life (Brown 1987; Bemporad and Romano 1993).

Susceptibility to psychological destabilization depends in part on *constitutional factors*, including genetic predisposition and personality (Andrews 1991; Enns and Cox 1997). However, the apparent epidemiological association of mental illness with female gender does not appear to have a biological basis, and may reflect differences in the life experiences of women and men (Bebbington 1988; Jenkins and Clare 1989).

Current psychosocial factors that seem to increase a person's vulnerability to destabilization are lack of social support, disharmony in intimate relationships, and *socioeconomic adversity* such as poor housing and unemployment (Brown 1987; Barnett and Gotlib 1988; Craig 1996). Conversely, friends, relatives and a supportive intimate relationship appear to be protective.

Stressors

Stressors are those factors that interact with a person's vulnerability to bring about psychological destabilization (Brown 1987). They include loss, the threat of loss, reminders of distressing experiences in the past, and physical illness. Losses, actual or threatened, are common accompaniments of many life events. Significantly, people who are already vulnerable to destabilization may also be at increased risk of experiencing negative life events (Brown 1987). What is important is not the event itself, but the way it is perceived and interpreted. The hypothesis that the threat of loss is associated with anxiety, while actual loss produces depression, is not fully supported by available research evidence (Goldberg and Huxley 1991). Part of the reason may be that people who are vulnerable to anxiety symptoms tend to pay selective attention to perceived threats (MacLeod 1991). Conversely, depression is associated with a tendency to focus on the negative aspects of experiences (Dalgleish and Watts 1990).

Reminders of distressing experiences in the past can be potent stressors (Brewin 1996). An apparently minor occurrence may be followed by psychological destabilization and a degree of emotional distress that is difficult to comprehend until the connection with the past is recognized. Several examples are given in Box 8.2.

Box 8.2   Reliving the past

A woman in her fifties felt panicky and tempted to run out
of the room whenever she lay down in a dentist's chair. She
was not particularly afraid of any pain that dental treatment
might cause, but explained that she felt powerless in the
chair. This recalled her feelings of powerlessness when she
was sexually assaulted as a child.

A man in his thirties developed severe depression with
ideas of worthlessness, and thoughts of suicide, following
a row at work with his manager. Although the issue had
been resolved, he subsequently dwelled on the idea that
he might have been fired, unable to find other work, and
consequently unable to provide adequately for his children.
His father had died when he was an infant, and his own
childhood had been spent in poverty.

A woman in her forties became profoundly depressed
following an argument with a female friend. There had been
no reconciliation, and the woman related the loss of her
friend to the death of her mother when she was a child.

Finally among the stressors, the strong association between
physical illness and psychological destabilization is well known
(Jorm 1995; Ustun and Sartorius 1995). While the causal relationships are complex, the research evidence shows clear benefit
from brief psychological interventions following the onset of acute
disease, and from pharmacotherapy for established depression,
even if this is 'understandable' in the light of the patient's coexisting physical disorder (Katon and Sullivan 1990; Guthrie 1996).

Symptom duration and restitution

The duration of symptoms following psychological destabilization depends on a range of factors (Goldberg and Huxley 1992).
Those that may lead to prolonged illness include lack of social

support, a dysfunctional intimate relationship, continuing socio-economic adversity, and chronic, disabling illness. In addition, secondary changes may inhibit recovery. For example, the person who increases his alcohol consumption to relieve anxiety symptoms is likely to find that his symptoms worsen after a binge, encouraging further excessive intake. Changes in family dynamics as a result of psychological symptoms can also encourage continuing illness, perhaps as a consequence of the mechanism of secondary gain (see Chapter 4).

Restitution refers to the process of losing symptoms. Symptoms may be lost as a result of recovered psychological stability, or as a consequence of neurotic coping mechanisms. Many anxiety disorders defined in psychiatry textbooks reflect neurotic coping. For example, the person with agoraphobia may never leave the house, and in consequence may gain substantial relief from his psychological symptoms.

Factors that appear to promote healthy recovery include a reduction in difficulties such as socioeconomic adversity or illness, and the occurrence of a fresh start event, such as the commencement of a new job or relationship (Brown 1987). In addition, a number of therapeutic approaches have been shown to be effective. It is to these that we now turn.

Approaches to management

A detailed account of the management of emotional and psychosocial problems would be out of place in this book. However, a number of issues are relevant to the aim of examining the consultation from a range of perspectives, and of identifying lessons for clinical practice.

Detection of distress

The first issue is that of detection. Most people who are psychologically distressed do not present to the doctor with explicit psychological difficulties, but in more subtle ways. Patients may communicate their distress through verbal or non-verbal cues, as discussed in Chapter 3. Davenport *et al.* (1987) found a strong correlation between patients' scores on a scale of psychological distress and the number of cues indicative of psychological disturbance that they gave during a consultation. Significantly, they also found that some doctors may behave in ways that enhance cue emission by the patient, while others may supress such emission. A subsequent study by Goldberg *et al.* (1993) showed that noticing and responding to verbal cues, making empathic comments and asking about feelings are all doctor behaviours that associated with an increased frequency of cue emission.

Patients may also give evidence of emotional distress through frequent consultations over apparently minor symptoms; through loss of control of chronic conditions such as asthma, diabetes or epilepsy; or through consultations about vague symptoms which do not reflect recognizable biophysical disease processes (Williams 1989). In addition, parents may present a child when the major problem lies elsewhere within the family (see Box 8.3).

The key to detection of psychological distress is empathic listening, discussed in Chapter 3. In addition, a number of screening instruments have been devised for use during the consultation. Although several of these instruments have been shown to

---

Box 8.3 The presenting child

A mother who regularly attended the practice with one or both of her two children presented with the 18-month-old who had two small pustules on his head. The child was not ill, and the doctor prescribed an anti-staphylococcal antibiotic. Three days later, the mother returned with the child and saw a different doctor. She explained that she was still worried about her son. The doctor examined the boy's head. The pustules were healing, and the boy was otherwise well. When he commented that she must have her hands full, coping with a toddler and a three-year-old, the child's mother started to cry and replied that everything would be all right if it was not for her partner (the child's father). It emerged that he was abusing her, that she did not know what to do, and that she was hoping the doctor could help her find a place in a women's refuge.

enhance detection rates, their routine use has not been shown to give measurable benefit in the screened population (Schade *et al.* 1998).

Working with the patient

Jaber *et al.* (1997) have listed three 'rules' that are implicit in many patient–doctor interactions with a disease focus, but which are decidedly unhelpful when consulting with a patient with psychosocial problems:

- The doctor is the expert.
- The doctor is the agent of change.
- The doctor's interpretation of the situation is sufficient to design a successful management plan.

Jaber and her colleagues, like other writers, suggest that it is more effective for the doctor to work *with* the patient in order to define and understand the nature and perceived causes of his distress, and to agree on an appropriate plan of management. The skills of active listening are important here, and are listed in Box 8.4. The aim is to elicit and agree with the patient an account of his emotional and psychosocial problems that provides an adequate basis for the joint development of a management plan. Sometimes a more directive approach to questioning is needed – when interviewing via an interpreter, for example. Some people are not comfortable talking about their feelings, and a focus on their behaviour in distressing situations may be more helpful. At times it may also be appropriate to check with the patient the legitimacy of the doctor's enquiries: 'Do you want to talk about this?' Patients have a right to privacy from their doctors, if they choose (see Chapter 3).

The doctor may also need to ask specific questions to screen for depressive symptoms, risk of self-harm, domestic violence, and excessive alcohol intake or recreational drug use. It is often helpful to ask about confiding relationships in the family and among the patient's friends and other contacts. If the patient is significantly depressed, it is important to ask about similar episodes in the past, their treatment and their resolution, and

---

Box 8.4   An incomplete list of the skills of active listening

- Using open questions, e.g. 'How have things been?'.
- Seeking elaboration, e.g. 'Tell me more about that'.
- Echoing, e.g. 'Not right since your mother died'.
- Uttering continuers, e.g. 'Go on'.
- Responding to verbal cues, e.g. 'You say you have been feeling pretty depressed recently'.
- Responding to non-verbal cues, e.g. 'You look very miserable'.
- Seeking clarification, e.g. 'Can you explain that to me?'.
- Seeking specific examples, e.g. 'Tell me about the last time this happened'.
- Exploring feelings, e.g. 'How did you feel about that?'.
- Empathic comments, e.g. 'I can see this is worrying you a great deal'.
- Legitimizing, e.g. 'I can understand how you would feel that way'.
- Summarizing, e.g. 'You were always close to your mother, and ever since she died you have been feeling unhappy in yourself, irritable with your family, and no longer interested in your work'.
- Scanning, e.g. 'Is there anything else?'.

---

precipitating factors for the current episode (Paykel and Priest 1992). Finally, elucidation of the patient's ideas, worries and wishes concerning management is important.

Developing a management plan

Each of us is different, with different past experiences, different aspirations and different issues in our lives that we need to address. There is no algorithm that the doctor can follow in consulting with a patient with psychological distress or psychosocial problems. Sometimes the very process of facilitating the patient in exploring his feelings and the problems in his life may provide an effective intervention. At other times, the doctor must work alongside the patient to develop a more action-based management plan. This may mean exploring the option of psychoactive medication, if an appropriate indication exists. The action plan may also include one or more of the following components:

- *Cognitive or behavioural interventions.* Formal cognitive-behaviour therapy is an effective treatment for many patients with psychological distress (Scott 1996; Harrington *et al.* 1998). It is too time-consuming for routine use in family practice, but a variety of brief interventions derived from the underlying theory are readily adapted to this setting (France and Robson 1997). However, good evidence for the effectiveness of such brief interventions is lacking at present.
- *Problem-solving treatment.* This is a structured approach to helping patients address practical and interpersonal problems in their lives. Intensive problem-solving therapy has been shown to be effective in the treatment of major depression and other disorders, but, like cognitive-behaviour therapy, is time-consuming as sole therapy (Mynors-Wallis 1996). However, the model is simple to learn, and is readily applied to specific practical and interpersonal problems in patients' lives (see Box 8.5).
- *Advocacy.* Advocacy on behalf of the patient or his family is an important role of the family doctor. There is a risk of encouraging dependency of course, and where possible patients should probably be supported in advocating for themselves. Occasionally the most valuable aspect of such support is the doctor's 'permission' to challenge authority. At other times, the relative authority of a telephone call or letter from the doctor is needed to encourage action by others.
- *Referral.* Referral to a psychiatrist should be considered if the patient has significant ideas of self-harm, is not responding to medication, has features of psychotic illness, or continues to be troubled by past experiences such as sexual abuse. Alternatively, referral to a clinical psychologist or social worker may be indicated. Interestingly, in one study, the outcomes of care of adult patients with major depression but without marked suicidal risk were similar whether they received care from their general practitioner, a psychiatrist (prescribing

Box 8.5 Problem-solving with patients

Problem-solving is a specific intervention aimed at helping patients to address practical and interpersonal issues in their lives. Examples might include the decision of where to live for a young person who wants to leave home, or the problem of dealing with unwanted sexual advances from a manager in the workplace. The role of the doctor is to facilitate the patient in thinking through and making his own decisions about such issues. The steps are as follows:

1 *Obtain a clear description of the problem from the patient.* If the patient has a number of problems, ask which is most pressing at the moment.
2 *Help the patient to define his goal.* For example: 'What would you like to be different from the way things are now?' Sometimes it is also useful to ask the patient to define an indicator of success: 'How will you know when things have changed?'
3 *Ask the patient to brainstorm actions that he might take to achieve this goal.* The key here is to focus on actions that the patient might take, not the things he would like others to do. Interrupt the patient from evaluating his ideas at this stage, and resist the temptation to give advice; the goal is to develop an action plan that is 'owned' by the patient. If the patient cannot think of any ideas, then arrange to see him again a few days later.
4 *Work through the ideas one by one, asking the patient to identify the advantages and disadvantages of each.* Again, it is the patient's views that are crucial.
5 *Ask the patient to select his preferred option, and then to identify the steps that he will need to take to implement this action plan.*
6 *'Stress inoculate'.* Ask the patient what would be the worst possible outcome as a result of his actions, and to brainstorm how he might cope with this. Once again, help the patient to work through his ideas, looking at the advantages and disadvantages of each, and to select his preferred option.

7 *Reassert your support for the patient, and arrange to see him again to discuss progress.*

Problem-solving in this way is not a complex process, and is easily taught to the patient. Indeed, patients may say that this is how they approach other issues in their lives, but that they had not thought to address their present problems in this way.

It is not a part of the process for the doctor to advise the patient on his possible options – something that distinguishes problem-solving for psychosocial issues from the management of physical disease. On occasion it may be appropriate to provide information that will help the patient to brainstorm his options. However, it is important not to influence the patient in making his own decisions.

A key step is ensuring that the patient has a clearly defined and measurable goal. Without this, the options that the patient identifies will lack focus, and may actually address a number of different goals. If the patient is not able to define a goal, then he is unlikely to develop and commit to a realistic action plan. In such cases it may be more appropriate to work with the patient in developing coping strategies. Useful approaches include:

- asking the patient to identify possible sources of help and support, and examining the advantages and disadvantages of these;
- enquiring about previous sources of support;
- offering empathy, legitimization of feelings, and an open door – 'I want you to let me know if I can help in any way'.

amitriptyline), a clinical psychologist (providing cognitive-behaviour therapy) or a social worker (providing counselling and case work). Social work was the treatment most positively evaluated by patients (Scott and Freeman 1992). In specific circumstances, referral to a drug and alcohol service, relationship counsellor, sexual violence unit or other specialist service may be appropriate.

Finally in this chapter, it is worth reiterating that attention to psychosocial issues is relevant to the care of all patients, not only those who present with emotional or interpersonal problems. All illness impacts on our perception of ourselves, on our behaviour, and on our family and other social interactions. The assessment and management of all patients should take into account the complex ways in which physical, psychological and social processes may interact.

9 ♦ Somatization and somatic fixation

If the common cold virus had not come into being on its own,
we would have been forced to invent it.

(Schild and Herman 1994: 34)

In 1995 the findings of the World Health Organization (WHO) Collaborative Study on psychological problems in primary health care were published (Ustun and Sartorius 1995). Adult patients presenting to family doctors or equivalent medical practitioners were recruited in centres across 14 countries. More than 25,000 participants were screened for psychological problems, and nearly 5500 were assessed in detail. The investigators concluded that psychological problems were common in all the settings examined in the study. On average, 24 per cent of participants had disorders that met diagnostic criteria for psychological conditions defined ICD-10 (WHO 1993). Amongst the most prevalent conditions in all centres were depressive disorders, anxiety disorders, alcohol use disorders and somatoform disorders. An additional 9 per cent of patients suffered from a 'subthreshold condition' that did not meet ICD-10 diagnostic criteria, but which was associated with significant distress and functional impairment. Although psychological *disorders* were commonly diagnosed by the researchers, psychological *problems* were given as the main reason for consulting by only 5.3 per cent of patients. In both developing and developed countries, most patients with defined psychological disorders presented with somatic complaints such as back pain, shortness of breath or dizziness.

In an earlier study, Bridges and Goldberg (1985) interviewed nearly 500 adult patients presenting with new episodes of illness to their general practitioners in Manchester, England. One-third of patients had psychiatric disorders, defined using the DSM-III classification (American Psychiatric Association 1980). Of these patients, 27 per cent had symptoms that were attributable to an accompanying physical disease, 17 per cent had no physical disease and presented with psychological symptoms, and 56 per cent presented with somatic symptoms for which no adequate physical cause could be identified.

It is clear from the findings of these studies, and from other research (Fabrega 1990; Barsky and Borus 1995) that psychological problems are common among people seeking primary medical care, but that the majority of psychologically distressed patients present with somatic symptoms even in the absence of coexisting physical disease.

The presentation of personal, emotional or social problems through somatic symptoms is called *somatization*. Not surprisingly, the tendency of patients to somatize is a major reason why doctors may fail to detect significant psychological distress (Goldberg and Bridges 1988). In this chapter I will review a number of hypotheses that seek to explain the phenomenon of somatization, and outline some approaches to classification and management. I will also discuss the trap of somatic fixation, into which doctors, patients and their families may all fall.

Somatizing patients

Why do patients somatize? A number of explanations have been advanced for the phenomenon of somatization. Pilowsky (1997) lists the following:

- *Presentation of the bodily changes that accompany emotional processes.* An example is the patient who hyperventilates when anxious, and then presents with dizzy spells (Gardner 1996).
- *The inability to express emotion.* It has been suggested that some people simply cannot express their feelings, a characteristic that has been labelled *alexithymia*, and that they therefore communicate distress in other ways (Sifneos 1996).

- *Excessive attention paid to bodily sensations,* which are then attributed to organic disease of some kind. Patients with irritable bowel syndrome may attribute their symptoms to serious bowel disease, even though they developed in the context of family problems or stress at work (Kettell *et al.* 1992).
- *Indirect communication of psychic pain,* perhaps using a modality that the patient learned within her family or other social group. Somatization may also provide an indirect way of communicating anger and dissatisfaction with others, including doctors and other health care professionals.
- *As an entry to the sick role.* As discussed in Chapter 1, the socially defined rights associated with sickness are more readily accessible to people with somatic symptoms than to those with mental symptoms.
- *As a response to the health care system.* This is discussed further in the section on somatic fixation below.

In addition, from a psychodynamic perspective, somatization may be seen as a defence, the primary gain of which is to prevent the patient from being overwhelmed by emotional distress. The process may be reinforced by secondary gains, such as relief from certain social expectations, or the receipt of sympathy from others (see Chapter 4).

Finally, the very notion of somatization may be a Western construct. In an analysis of the language of emotion in different cultures, Mumford (1993) identified three basic modes of expression: somatic sensations, somatic metaphor and abstract psychological language. People whose first language lacks specific words for depression or anxiety may have no means of describing psychological distress except in somatic terms.

Somatization classified

Blacker (1991) has suggested a useful classification, grouping somatizing patients into three categories:

- disguisers;
- deniers;
- don't knows.

Patients classified by Blacker as *disguisers* recognize that they have a psychological or psychosocial problem, but use a physical complaint as a 'ticket of admission' to gain access to the doctor (see Box 3.2). *Deniers*, in contrast, tend to resist discussion and exploration of emotional or psychosocial issues, and often develop chronic somatic illnesses. This category includes patients with the somatoform disorders described in ICD-10 and DSM-IV (WHO 1992; American Psychiatric Association 1994). *Don't knows* are aware of their emotional or social problems but present with somatic symptoms, and are worried that these may reflect physical disease.

Although the categories in this simple classification are not completely watertight, it does have some support in published research (Bridges and Goldberg 1985). Furthermore, the classification provides a guide to management.

Management of somatic symptoms

Patients who are 'disguisers' and 'don't knows' in Blacker's classification usually present with a relatively short history, either of new symptoms or of exacerbation of a more chronic physical problem. The key to helping these patients lies in detecting the possibility of psychological or psychosocial difficulties, and in opening up the agenda of the consultation to include discussion of emotional and psychosocial issues. A clinical example is given in Box 9.1 to illustrate the process, and a management approach developed by Goldberg and others is described below.

The patient described in Box 9.1 would be included in the group of 'Don't knows' in Blacker's classification. Identification and discussion of the psychosocial aspects of her illness allowed the patient and doctor to agree on a possible link with her somatic symptoms, and to negotiate an appropriate management plan that took into account both biophysical and psychosocial elements.

Patients in the category of 'disguisers' will be familiar to every doctor who has heard the words 'By the way, doctor, while I am here'. The consultation described in Box 8.3 gave an example in which a child's illness was presented as the 'ticket'. Some patients, of course, 'disguise' their psychosocial reasons for consulting,

---

Box 9.1   Work stress presenting as irritable bowel syndrome

For many years, a 32-year-old female school teacher had experienced intermittent constipation associated with colicky abdominal pain. She presented to her family doctor with a six-week history of exacerbation of both these symptoms. The patient had not previously sought help for her abdominal problems, which were consistent with a diagnosis of irritable bowel syndrome (Maxwell *et al.* 1997). The doctor asked if she had any thoughts about what might have exacerbated her symptoms, and the patient replied that she had been under a lot of stress at school recently. However, she was worried that her symptoms might reflect bowel cancer or other serious organic problem. The patient described no alarm symptoms such as recent weight loss, and physical examination was unremarkable. Further discussion of the patient's history demonstrated a clear association between episodes of stress in her life and exacerbation of her bowel symptoms. The patient and doctor agreed that this was the most likely explanation for the current problem, but that the doctor would arrange appropriate investigations to exclude other possible disease. In the meantime, the patient decided to accept the stressful situation at work, which she felt would resolve itself over the next few weeks. She also wanted symptomatic relief of her colic, and her doctor prescribed an antispasmodic and advised reduction in caffeine intake.

---

but also 'don't know' if they should be concerned about their somatic symptoms.

Reattribution of symptoms

Goldberg *et al.* (1989) have described a useful approach to consultations with patients who are thought to be somatizing, and who fall into either of the categories of 'disguisers' or 'don't knows'. The model has three stages:

1 feeling understood;
2 changing the agenda;
3 making the link.

Feeling understood reflects the need and expectation that we all have when we visit the doctor, that he should listen to us and take our complaints seriously. In addition to those rapport-building behaviours that were discussed in Chapter 3, it is important for the doctor to take a full history of the presenting symptom, to elicit associated symptoms, and to explore the patient's explanatory model for her illness. It is also important to respond to emotional cues, and if necessary to probe the patient's mood state with a question such as 'Apart from the pain, how have you been feeling in yourself?'. Relevant social and family factors should be explored, and in general the aim is to discuss both biophysical and psychosocial factors as they arise. An appropriately focused physical examination is most important, even if the doctor does not expect to find any abnormalities.

The next step, *changing the agenda*, is predicated on the assumption that the doctor is content that no significant disease process explains the patient's symptoms. Goldberg and colleagues recommend feeding back to the patient a brief summary of the doctor's findings on physical examination, acknowledging the reality of the patient's symptoms, and then tentatively linking them to life events or the patient's mood state. For example:

> You have told me that your headaches have become more severe and more frequent over the last few months. I was not able to find any cause for them when I examined you, but I was struck that you have been feeling pretty down and tearful since your mother died, and the headaches also got worse since then.

Making the link describes the process of strengthening the patient's *reattribution* of her symptoms from a physical cause to a psychosocial association. Several strategies are suggested. These include giving explanations based on psychophysiological processes (Salmon *et al.* 1999). For example:

> When people get upset they tend to tense the muscles in their bodies. If the muscles stay tense for a long time they

start to ache. The headaches that you have been getting are typical of the pain that comes from tension in the muscles of the head and neck.

Other strategies include engaging the patient in a thought experiment (for example, asking her to imagine carrying a heavy suitcase, as a demonstration of how muscles ache when tense) and exploring examples of somatization within the patient's family of origin. For example, if the doctor has learned that the patient's mother also suffered frequent headaches, then it may be useful to ask a question such as 'What sort of situations used to bring on your mother's headaches?'. Somatizing behaviour is frequently learned in the patient's family of origin.

Of course, the doctor's job does not end with an agreement to reattribute the patient's symptoms to psychosocial processes. He may have elicited features suggestive of a depressive illness or other psychiatric disorder, for which treatment may need to be negotiated. He may also need to work with the patient in addressing family, social or other problems (see Chapter 8).

One criticism of the model described by Goldberg and his colleagues has been that the doctor may detect significant psychosocial problems, which could account for the patient's somatic symptoms, but he may not be fully confident that somatization is the full explanation. To return to the example in Box 9.1, the patient may have developed a rectal carcinoma at a young age. The key to developing a management plan is that the patient's symptoms do not have to be attributed from the outset *either* to biophysical disease *or* to psychosocial problems. A tentative link can be discussed with the patient, and psychosocial issues addressed, while further investigations are undertaken. More recent descriptions of the Goldberg reattribution model have changed the second step to *broadening the agenda* (Gask 1995).

Managing chronic somatization ('deniers')

The approach outlined above for the management of acute somatization can be positively unhelpful in consultations with chronic somatizers, who by definition resist exploration of emotional and psychosocial issues. McDaniel *et al.* (1989) have described a useful alternative, based on the biopsychosocial model that was described in Chapter 7. They suggest a number of principles to guide the doctor in his interactions with a somatizing patient. These include the following:

- *From the beginning, pay attention to both biomedical and psychosocial elements of the problem.* Questions such as 'What does your partner think is wrong with you?' or 'Has anyone in your family suggested a particular treatment for you?' allow the doctor to demonstrate a concern for the psychosocial context of the patient's illness, and to avoid an exclusive focus on its somatic aspects, without asking directly about feelings and relationships.
- *Solicit information about the patient's symptoms, but do not let this information run the interview.* Throughout our medical training, we learn to focus our questions and attention on those aspects of the patient's story that are of greatest help in arriving at a differential diagnosis, and in distinguishing between the various diagnostic hypotheses (Gale and Marsden 1983). This approach to interviewing clearly has its place, but does little to demonstrate understanding to the patient who is trying to communicate her distress through somatic symptoms. Active listening is the key here, and it is often helpful to seek precise descriptions of vague symptoms, and for episodic symptoms, to ask about particular episodes. For example: 'When did you last have one of these dizzy spells? What were you doing at the time? Can you describe what happened, from beginning to end? Did you notice anything else?' It is also important to ask about the social context: 'Who else was there? What did they say? What did you think of that?' For more continuous symptoms, it can be helpful to take the patient through a typical day in her life. Frequent summaries of what the patient has said can be helpful in demonstrating that the doctor has been paying attention, in checking that he has understood the patient's story so far, and in moving the interview on to further aspects of the patient's story.
- *Develop a collaborative relationship with the patient.* Describing symptoms as mysterious and baffling, but indicating a desire to collaborate with the patient in understanding them further, and in helping her to cope with the associated disability, can

be instrumental in developing a working relationship that is based on a spirit of mutual enquiry. The aim, over time, is to develop a shared explanatory model of the patient's illness that is accepted as valid by both patient and doctor.

- *See the patient at regular intervals, not just when symptoms occur or intensify.* This conveys the doctor's ongoing concern for the patient, and may also allow discussion of the patient's symptoms when they are absent or less severe. At such times, the patient may be more willing to discuss possible emotional or social factors.

- *Encourage the patient to see only one doctor in the practice, and discourage visits to other health care providers, except following specific referral.* Unwitting statements and actions by other health professionals may seriously undermine the patient's trust in her primary doctor, and in the development of mutual understanding between them. Care by multiple providers can also lead to the situation described by Balint (1986) as *collusion of anonymity*, in which a number of people are providing care, but none accepts ultimate responsibility for the outcome of that care. Box 9.2 gives an example of the harm that can result.

- *Elicit the patient's and family's understanding of the problem.* The importance of exploring the patient's understanding of her illness, her fears and associated expectations of the doctor, was discussed in detail in Chapter 2. Questions about the family's views can also be tremendously valuable in explaining the patient's illness (Mauksch and Roesler 1990).

- *Elicit recent life events and ask about any associated worsening in symptoms.* Such questions can demonstrate concern about psychosocial issues affecting the patient, and may raise the possibility of a link in the patient's mind, but avoid the doctor having to make a firm declaration of his own thoughts. For example: 'You mentioned earlier that your mother died two years ago, and that you were very close. I was wondering if your back pain got any worse after that?'.

- *Ask about, and constantly return to, the patient's strengths and areas of competence.* An awareness of oneself as capable of competent action in some area of one's life appears to be important for coping with illness and other adversity (Beardslee 1989).

- *Avoid psychosocial fixation.* This is a common trap for the doctor. We are all at risk of serious disease, and patients who somatize are no exception. It is important that the doctor remains alert to this possibility, and assesses all symptoms with the possibility in mind. The art is to consider and address biomedical and psychosocial issues concurrently.

• *Find a way to enjoy working with patients who somatize.* Epithets such as 'heartsink' not only are unprofessional (Pilowsky 1997) but also reinforce negative feelings on the part of the doctor. Yet such patients often feel frustrated, angry at the medical establishment, and discouraged about their illness. Strategies for developing a more positive relationship include: identifying and noting things about the patient that command respect; listening to the patient's symptoms as metaphors for wider problems; discussing the case with another doctor in the practice; and sharing the patient's care with a psychiatrist or other mental health professional. Two randomized control trials in the United States have shown that a single psychiatric consultation for patients presenting to family practitioners with chronic somatization may reduce their health care charges (a crude measure of health service use) and improve physical function, without any change in health status or satisfaction with care (Smith *et al.* 1986; 1995).

• *Judge progress in these patients by monitoring changes in their level of functioning, rather than in their symptoms.* Patients who have somatized their distress for many years, often since childhood, rarely lose their symptoms completely. More realistic goals involve an increase in functioning in areas such as work and family relationships.

Somatic fixation

Most definitions of somatization reflect an understanding of the phenomenon as something that occurs within the psyche of the individual patient (Pilowsky 1997). An alternative view regards somatization as a manifestation of the process of *somatic fixation*, 'that phenomenon by which, as a result of continuously one-sided emphasis on the somatic aspects of diseases, complaints, or problems, people become more and more entangled in and increasingly dependent on the medical apparatus' (van Eijk *et al.* 1983: 6). All illnesses have physical, psychological and social

---

Box 9.2 Collusion of anonymity

A 23-year-old woman gave a three-year history of episodic central abdominal pain that remained unexplained despite intensive investigation by her general practitioner. The woman discussed with friends the temporal association of her pain with the ups and downs of her family and private life, and expressed the idea that her pain might in some way be caused by things that upset her. Her general practitioner discounted this possibility, and referred her to a surgeon. The surgeon arranged more tests, the results of which proved normal. He then undertook an exploratory laparotomy 'to check that he had not missed anything' before discharging the woman back to the care of her general practitioner.

   This woman underwent unnecessary surgery because her general practitioner had made what was essentially a defensive referral, to protect himself against the remote possibility that he had failed to detect significant organic pathology. The surgeon saw his role entirely in terms of treating or excluding such pathology, and believed responsibility for psychosocial issues to lie with the general practitioner. Neither doctor was willing to shoulder responsibility for the overall health and well-being of the patient. Following her operation, the woman continued to experience abdominal pain at particularly stressful and painful times in her life.

---

aspects. Somatic fixation occurs when the doctor, patient or family focuses exclusively on the physical elements.

It has been hypothesized by various authors that somatic fixation may be initiated or reinforced at the very first consultation concerning an episode of illness (McDaniel *et al.* 1989; Schild and Herman 1994). Rather than listen to the psychosocial aspects of the patient's story, the doctor concentrates exclusively on the somatic. He asks only about physical symptoms, ignores psychosocial cues, and may arrange investigations to exclude organic disease. If these give positive results, then treatment focuses on correcting the biological abnormality. If negative, more

---

Box 9.3   An example of somatic fixation

A 32-year-old man presented to his family doctor
complaining of pain and tiredness in his neck, especially
at the end of the working day. The doctor could find no
specific abnormalities on physical examination and arranged
for X-rays of the cervical spine. These appeared normal.
He subsequently referred the patient to an occupational
physician and a neurologist. Neither specialist could provide
a physical diagnosis. Finally, the general practitioner asked
the patient if he thought that his symptoms might be related
to work stress or family problems. The patient expressed
anger at these suggestions and said that he was sure that the
doctors were all missing the diagnosis. He never consulted
the general practitioner again.

---

investigations may be ordered, the patient referred for a specialist opinion, or a placebo prescribed (Straus and Cavanaugh 1996).
Either way, the patient's attribution of her illness to physical
causes is reinforced. If her symptoms fail to resolve, the doctor
may raise with her the possibility of a psychological cause. It is
far too late by now, of course, and the patient is likely to feel
angry and confused. She may reject the doctor's suggestion completely, and adhere ever more firmly to a physical attribution of
her illness (see Box 9.3).

   The process of somatic fixation can occur even when the
patient's symptoms are clearly the result of organic pathology.
There is evidence that psychological stress may predispose to the
development of infection, and possibly other diseases (Biondi
and Zannino 1997). Furthermore, given the development of a
symptomatic disease process, people are more likely to seek medical attention if they are psychologically distressed than if they
are not (Cohen and Williamson 1991). The doctor may concen-
trate on the disease process alone, but this may not be the best
approach for the patient (see Box 9.4 for a tragic illustration).

   Somatic fixation may also occur in chronic illness. Sometimes
it is the patient who fixates on her somatic problems, perhaps
for reasons of secondary gain (see Chapter 4), and the doctor

---

Box 9.4   A tragic outcome

A 23-year-old man split up with his partner of five years.
A few days later he developed diarrhoea and vomiting, and
called his general practitioner. The doctor attended him at
home and diagnosed viral gastroenteritis. The patient made
no mention of the recent events in his life, and the doctor
attributed the patient's apparent distress to his gastrointestinal
illness. The doctor gave the patient an intramuscular
injection of prochlorperazine, and left. A few hours later
the patient hanged himself.

---

may collude with this. The epidemiological association between
chronic illness and psychological distress, particularly depression, is well known (Jorm 1995; Ustun and Sartorius 1995).
Furthermore, there is evidence that treatment of psychological
comorbidity in disabling illness is associated with an improved
patient outcome (see Chapter 8). Failure to address psychosocial
problems associated with chronic physical illness may mean that
opportunities to intervene and improve function are missed.

Conclusion

Family doctors clearly have a considerable opportunity to prevent the development of somatic fixation in their day-to-day
clinical practice. During the 1970's, members of the Institute of
General Practice at the University of Nijmegen, Netherlands,
undertook a series of studies into the process of somatic fixation.
This work was summarized in a book *To Heal or to Harm* (Grol
1983), much of which remains relevant today. In their book, the
authors emphasize the importance of establishing and maintaining rapport with the patient; of paying detailed attention to both
somatic and psychosocial issues; and of managing psychosocial
and somatic problems concurrently and with equal competence.
These principles provide a succinct summary of the approaches
discussed in this chapter.

The consultation back in context

... a useful person to have as a fellow traveller; able when necessary to help with the navigation or repair the engine, but mostly there to share the experience and help to reflect on it. He doesn't know, any more than the patient, how or where the journey will end; he is also on a journey of his own.

(John Salinsky 1987: 88)

In this book I have tried to examine the consultation from a number of perspectives, focusing on relevant research and its implications for practice. In this final chapter I want to locate the individual consultation in the context of the ongoing patient–doctor relationship. When a patient consults a doctor for the first time, he initiates a conversation that has the potential to continue until one or the other dies. The doctor, on seeing the patient, accepts a responsibility that extends well beyond the here and now of the single interaction. This raises a number of issues which I will discuss under three headings:

- prevention;
- continuity;
- the purpose of the consultation.

Prevention

Prevention lies at the heart of primary health care. Every consultation, and every action of the doctor within each consultation, should reflect a concern to empower the patient, and to maximize his present and future choices. Usually this is achieved through attempts to prevent diseases that the patient does not yet have, to detect and treat asymptomatic conditions, and to reduce the current and future disability resulting from existing illness: primary, secondary and tertiary prevention, respectively. Rather than attempt a detailed review of strategies for preventive care in general practice, I want to highlight some issues concerning primary and secondary prevention that seem particularly relevant to the individual consultation, but which are not always addressed in standard texts (e.g. Rose 1992).

Primary prevention

Many of the factors that influence health are outside the control of the individual doctor in her practice, although this does not absolve doctors from a responsibility to speak out and to advocate for the communities whom they serve (Heath 1998). Within the consultation, the commonest opportunities for primary prevention are through immunization and lifestyle advice. Practices need information management systems that record immunizations given, recall patients when they are next due, and prompt the doctor to offer immunizations that are overdue when the patient consults about another issue.

Many aspects of lifestyle affect health. Perhaps those most commonly discussed with doctors are smoking and drinking, other recreational drug use, diet, exercise, sexual behaviour and injury prevention. Ashenden *et al.* (1997) undertook a systematic review of studies of the effectiveness of lifestyle interventions in general practice. They found that while many interventions had some impact, most had, at best, a moderate effect. Furthermore, while much research on lifestyle advice has studied the effectiveness of interventions in changing patients' behaviour, relatively few studies have also assessed health outcomes.

While few would dispute that family doctors have a responsibility to advise patients of their health risks, and to support them in developing a healthier lifestyle, there are dangers in doing this unthinkingly and without careful reflection (Sullivan 1995). It would be crass, for example, to raise the issue of smoking behaviour during a consultation about problems in a person's

---

Box 10.1 The transtheoretical model of change

This is a useful model for understanding the process of behaviour change, and for tailoring interventions to the situation of the individual patient (Prochaska *et al.* 1992). The transtheoretical model summarizes research on how people change their behaviour into five stages:

- *Precontemplation*. The person does not intend to change, either because they do not know the risks of their present behaviour, or in spite of knowing the risks.
- *Contemplation*. The person intends to change, but has not yet started to do so.
- *Preparation*. The person is actively planning to change.
- *Action*. The person is making changes in their behaviour.
- *Maintenance*. The person has changed behaviour, and is taking steps to sustain this and to resist the temptation to relapse.

In this model, people progress from one stage to the next, but may relapse at any stage. Indeed, relapse is seen as a natural part of the change process, and provides an opportunity for the person to learn and to explore other ways of changing lifestyle habits.

The value of the transtheoretical model is that it not only identifies stages in the process of change, but also provides a guide for intervention that is tailored to the patient, and may be more effective than an approach that is the same for all patients (Prochaska *et al.* 1994). Thus, a patient in the precontemplation stage may benefit most from information and other interventions that aim at consciousness-raising. For example, a person who smokes may be asked if he has ever considered stopping, and perhaps be offered a health education booklet outlining the risks of continuing.

A person who is contemplating stopping smoking can be helped to explore the pros and cons of continuing, and the doctor could feed back observations about how smoking is already affecting the patient's health. For example: 'I notice that you have had several episodes of bronchitis in the last two years. I am sure you don't want me to lecture you, but I do think that your bronchitis is an early sign of the

---

damage that cigarette smoking is doing to your lungs. If we ignore this early sign, I am really concerned that your health is going to get a lot worse over the next five years.'

A patient who is preparing for change needs help and encouragement. A smoker may benefit from advice to throw out cigarettes, lighters and ashtrays, or support in examining alternatives to a cigarette after meals. Encouragement and support need to continue throughout the action phase and into that of maintenance. The patient may also be asked to identify the benefits that he has noticed from the change, and to discuss ways of coping in times of temptation.

The transtheoretical model has application to facilitating change in all behaviour, not just smoking. Sometimes the patient will proceed through several stages in one consultation. At other times, a person will stay in one stage for months or years. Relapses can provide opportunities to learn, and the doctor can help the patient to examine what went wrong, and how he could overcome this in future.

One limitation of the transtheoretical model is that it deals largely with the psychology of the individual. Much behaviour both reflects and contributes to social processes involving others. These social processes can make individual change extremely difficult. For example, a smoker's partner may also smoke, and she may resent the loss of ten minutes enjoying a cigarette together over coffee. Attempts to help patients address health-damaging behaviour may be far more successful if the social barriers to change are identified and addressed.

primary emotional relationship. More worryingly, Butler *et al.* (1998) have reported that smokers may occasionally fail to seek necessary medical attention because they fear that the doctor will lecture them. The researchers conducted qualitative interviews with smokers and ex-smokers, and concluded that smoking interventions which patients found acceptable took account of their receptiveness at the time; were conveyed in a respectful tone; avoided preaching; showed support and caring; and attempted to understand the patient as a unique individual. A useful approach to tailoring lifestyle interventions to the situation of the individual patient is outlined in Box 10.1.

Secondary prevention

Secondary prevention is the detection and treatment of disease before it becomes clinically manifest. There are two main approaches to secondary prevention: systematic screening and opportunistic case finding. Screening programmes have conventionally been assessed using criteria based on those of Wilson and Jungner (1968). A more recent approach has been to compare directly the costs, benefits and other outcomes of screening and of not screening (Kerr 1998). The implementation of a screening programme at practice level requires an information management system, and systems for data entry, monitoring and recall. The information management system should also prompt the doctor that a screening procedure is due when the patient consults about another matter.

Case finding is opportunistic screening in the consultation. A combination of patient recall and case finding during consultations is probably the most effective way of achieving a high uptake of population screening in general practice (Hart *et al.* 1991; van der Weijden and Grol 1998). Screening and case finding may, however, carry risks for the individual even when they have been evaluated and shown to be beneficial at the population level. A study by Haynes *et al.* (1978) demonstrated that among steelworkers who were newly identified as hypertensive, illness-related absence from work increased substantially. This research prompted the *labelling hypothesis*, that information about unfavourable risk factors may reduce health status, even in the absence of demonstrable pathology. Importantly, further studies have suggested that adequate counselling and follow-up may reduce the adverse impact of labelling on health (Lefebvre *et al.* 1988).

A second potentially detrimental effect of screening is that people who engage in risky behaviour but who screen negative on some test may take this as evidence for the safety of their lifestyle. This has been called the *certificate of health* effect (Tymstra and Bieleman 1987). Indeed, although it has been contested, there is some evidence that people who have screened negative may actually increase their risk-taking behaviour, perhaps consequent on a false sense of immunity (Otten *et al.* 1993). The implications for post-test counselling are clear.

Continuity

The provision of 'personal, primary and continuing medical care to individuals and families' has long been held as a defining characteristic of good general practice (Royal College of General Practitioners 1972: 1). And yet, factors that include changes in the structure and organization of general practice, the growth of consumerism, and increasing mobility of patients, have reduced the likelihood of a long-term relationship between patient and doctor (Baker 1997). Does this matter? There is clear evidence of an association between continuity of care and the quality of that care, as measured by the amount of preventive activity undertaken, the recognition of psychosocial problems, the number and duration of hospital admissions, and levels of patient and doctor satisfaction (Freeman and Hjortdahl 1997; Bowman and Nicklin 1998). However, the existence of an association does not imply causality. If there is a causal relationship, it is probably bidirectional: continuity of care leading to increased satisfaction, and satisfaction with care making the patient more likely to consult the same doctor again in the future. Furthermore, while continuity may be a prerequisite for the development of a personal relationship between patient and doctor, it cannot guarantee the quality of that relationship.

Freeman and Hjortdahl (1997) have attempted to resolve some of this confusion by distinguishing between two types of continuity: longitudinal and personal. *Longitudinal* continuity they define as care given by one doctor over a period of time. *Personal* continuity is an ongoing therapeutic relationship between patient and doctor, persisting even if the patient sees other practitioners on occasion. The nature and quality of contacts is more important than their number, and the patient will typically see 'his doctor' as their most valued source of care. Longitudinal continuity is more easily measured, but personal continuity may be more clinically relevant.

How can personal continuity be fostered at the level of the individual consultation, and what are its implications? The importance of demonstrating empathy, trustworthiness and respect for the patient were discussed in Chapter 3. Adequate clinical records are similarly important, as are clear arrangements for appropriate follow-up and review. Even when care has been sought for a single episode of illness, a plan should be negotiated for review if the patient does not recover as expected. Attention to issues of prevention and health promotion reflect a concern for the whole patient, with a whole life to lead.

Continuity of care provides the doctor with the opportunity to use *time* as an instrument of diagnosis and management. This is the case far more in family practice than in specialist or hospital practice. Much of the illness presenting in community settings is self-limiting. If the doctor is confident that serious illness has been excluded, then negotiating with the patient to await events may provide the most appropriate management of an individual illness episode. Such negotiation may also provide opportunities for discussion of help-seeking behaviour.

Time and personal continuity also provide the family doctor with opportunities to intervene in chronic problems and difficulties. There is evidence, for example, that it may be more useful to raise the issue of quitting with a smoker when he presents with smoking-related symptoms rather than at other times (Stott and Pill 1990). Many psychosocial problems, and much dysfunctional illness behaviour, are maintained by unhelpful family dynamics that can be hard for the patient to modify or for the doctor to challenge (see Chapters 7 and 9). Sometimes, the best opportunity to help is at times of crisis. An important skill in family practice lies in knowing when to keep silent, and when to intervene.

The purpose of the consultation

Much of this book has been concerned with issues of the *how* of consulting, while issues concerning *why* have been relegated to a justifying role. I have paid little attention to questions about the fundamental purpose of the consultation: why has the social institution of the consultation been created, and why does it persist? What is its social and personal value? Exploring these questions in detail could fill several more volumes, but in this final section I want to reflect on two essays by general practitioners that draw together many of the themes of this book.

In his monograph, *Feasible Socialism*, Julian Tudor Hart (1994) describes the consultation as an opportunity for the coproduction of health. He points out that both diagnosis and treatment depend on the active involvement of the patient as well as that of the doctor. The consultation has social value as an arena in which patient and doctor work closely together in order to enhance the former's health. Hart goes on to suggest that recognition of patients as coproducers rather than consumers of health care 'would begin to solve several problems which are otherwise likely to get worse. As co-producers, patients must share much more actively both in defining their problems and in devising feasible solutions, than they have in the past' (Hart 1994: 43). From this perspective, patient and doctor come to the consultation with differing knowledge and skills, but with equal status as workers. If they are to be effective in their work, each must value and respect the contribution of the other.

While Hart's focus is on the consultation as a unit of production, that of Iona Heath (1995) is on the contribution that general practice makes to the individual and society. She sees the generalism of family practice as far more radical than a mere concern with the diagnosis and management of a range and variety of human disease, important and challenging though these activities are:

> All aspects of human existence are legitimate concerns of the general practitioner provided that they are presented as a problem by the patient. This means that the general practitioner is obliged to deal with the complexity of each individual patient and should never be content to respond to a patient by saying 'That's not my business or my problem'.
>
> (Heath 1995: 26)

Heath identifies two key roles of the general practitioner: 'firstly to serve as interpreter and guardian at the interface between illness and disease; and secondly to serve as a witness to the patient's experience of illness and disease' (Heath 1995: 26). The role of interpreter and guardian at the interface between illness and disease is both technical and human. On the one hand, the doctor's technical training is what enables her to recognize, label and treat disease. On the other, her awareness of herself as a fellow human is her greatest asset in recognizing and interpreting the distress of illness:

As doctors, we combine the subjective experience of our own bodies and minds, with the objective theoretical understanding of the science of their working. By straddling this divide within his or her own body, the generalist doctor is qualified to interpret the interface between illness and disease.

(Heath 1995: 28)

The development of bodily empathy with the patient provides the basis for the doctor's second role, that of witness to the patient's experience of illness. We need to communicate our distress to others, and to engage in dialogue with them, if we are to make sense of our experiences and of how we respond. Without such witnessing, 'the individual and collective experience of illness and disease is harsher and more lonely, and humanity is the meaner' (Heath 1995: 30).

I think I agree with the conclusions of these two writers. Both emphasize the importance for good family practice of the interaction between patient and doctor. I started this book with a quotation asserting that general practice is the easiest discipline in medicine to practise badly, and the most difficult to do well. The challenge of doing general practice well is that it demands not only a high level of technical knowledge and skill, but also considerable interpersonal competence and self-knowledge. It requires commitment to the community served, with a willingness to form ongoing relationships with patients and families, to develop awareness of local cultural issues, and to learn continually from the experience. Every consultation provides the doctor with a test of that learning, and with an opportunity to further it.

References

Altschuler, J. (1997) *Working with Chronic Illness*. Basingstoke: Macmillan.

American Psychiatric Association (1980) *Diagnostic and Statistical Manual of Mental Disorders: Third Edition (DSM-III)*. Washington, DC: American Psychiatric Association.

American Psychiatric Association (1994) *Diagnostic and Statistical Manual of Mental Disorders: Fourth Edition (DSM-IV)*. Washington, DC: American Psychiatric Association.

Anderson, R. (1987) The unremitting burden on carers, *British Medical Journal*, 294: 73–4.

Andrews, G. (1991) Anxiety, personality and anxiety disorders, *International Review of Psychiatry*, 3: 293–302.

Argyle, M. (1994) *The Psychology of Interpersonal Behaviour*. London: Penguin.

Ashenden, R., Silagy, C. and Weller, D. (1997) A systematic review of the effectiveness of promoting lifestyle change in general practice, *Family Practice*, 14: 160–76.

Baker, R. (1997) Will the future GP remain a personal doctor? *British Journal of General Practice*, 47: 831–4.

Balint, E. (1973) The 'flash' technique – its freedom and its discipline, in E. Balint and J.S. Norell (eds), *Six Minutes for the Patient*. London: Tavistock Publications.

Balint, M. (1973) Research in psychotherapy, in E. Balint and J.S. Norell (eds), *Six Minutes for the Patient*. London: Tavistock Publications.

Balint, M. (1986) *The Doctor, His Patient and the Illness*. Edinburgh: Churchill Livingstone.

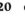

Balint, E. and Norell, J.S. (eds) (1973) *Six Minutes for the Patient*. London: Tavistock Publications.

Barkham, M. (1988) Empathy in counselling and psychotherapy: present status and future directions, *Counselling Psychology Quarterly*, 1: 407–28.

Barnett, P.A. and Gotlib, I.H. (1988) Psychosocial functioning and depression, *Psychological Bulletin*, 104: 97–126.

Barsky, A.J. and Borus, J.F. (1995) Somatization and medicalization in the era of managed care, *Journal of the American Medical Association*, 274: 1931–4.

Beardslee, W.R. (1989) The role of self-understanding in resilient individuals, *American Journal of Orthopsychiatry*, 59: 266–78.

Bebbington, P.E. (1998) Sex and depression, *Psychological Medicine*, 28: 1–8.

Beckman, H.B. and Frankel, R.M. (1984) The effect of physician behavior on the collection of data, *Annals of Internal Medicine*, 101: 692–6.

Bemporad, J.R. and Romano, S. (1993) Childhood experience and adult depression: a review of studies, *American Journal of Psychoanalysis*, 53: 301–15.

Bendix, T. (1982) *The Anxious Patient*. Edinburgh: Churchill Livingstone.

Berne, E. (1961) *Transactional Analysis in Psychotherapy*. New York: Grove Press.

Berne, E. (1964) *Games People Play*. New York: Grove Press.

Berne, E. (1972) *What Do You Say after You Say Hello?* New York: Grove Press.

Biondi, M. and Zannino, L.G. (1997) Psychological stress, neuroimmunomodulation, and susceptibility to infectious diseases in animals and man: a review, *Psychotherapy and Psychosomatics*, 66: 3–26.

Blacker, R. (1991) The diagnosis of patients at risk of psychiatric disorder, in R. Corney (ed.), *Developing Communication and Counselling Skills in Medicine*. London: Tavistock/Routledge.

Blaxter, M. (1983) The causes of disease. Women talking, *Social Science and Medicine*, 17: 59–69.

Blaxter, M. and Paterson, E. (1982) *Mothers and Daughters. A Three-Generation Study of Health Attitudes and Behaviour*. London: Heinemann.

Bowman, M.A. and Nicklin, D.E. (1998) New developments in family medicine, *Journal of the American Medical Association*, 279: 1437–8.

Brewin, C.R. (1996) Cognitive processing of adverse experiences, *International Review of Psychiatry*, 8: 333–9.

Bridges, K.W. and Goldberg, D.P. (1985) Somatic presentation of DSM III psychiatric disorders in primary care, *Journal of Psychosomatic Research*, 29: 563–9.

Bridges-Webb, C. (1966) General practice in Australia from 1788 to 1990: a personal commentary, in *General Practice in Australia: 1996.* Canberra: Commonwealth Department of Health and Family Services.

Brody, H. (1994) 'My story is broken; can you help me fix it?' Medical ethics and the joint construction of narrative, *Literature and Medicine,* 13: 79–92.

Brothers, L. (1989) A biological perspective on empathy, *American Journal of Psychiatry,* 146: 10–19.

Brown, G.W. (1987) Social factors and the development and course of depressive disorders in women, *British Journal of Social Work,* 17: 615–34.

Brown, G.W. and Harris, T.O. (1978) *Social Origins of Depression.* London: Tavistock.

Brown, J., Stewart, M., McCracken, E., McWhinney, I.R. and Levenstein, J. (1986) The patient-centred clinical method. 2. Definition and application, *Family Practice,* 3: 75–9.

Buetow, S.A. (1995) What do general practitioners and their patients want from general practice and are they receiving it? A framework, *Social Science and Medicine,* 40: 213–21.

Butler, C.C., Pill, R. and Stott, N.C.H. (1998) Qualitative study of patients' perceptions of doctors' advice to quit smoking: implications for opportunistic health promotion, *British Medical Journal,* 316: 1878–81.

Byrne, P.S. and Long, B.E.L. (1976) *Doctors Talking to Patients.* London: Her Majesty's Stationary Office.

Cameron, D. (1985) *Feminism and Linguistic Theory.* London: Macmillan.

Charles, C., Gafni, A. and Whelan, T. (1997) Shared decision-making in the medical encounter: what does it mean? (or it takes at least two to tango), *Social Science and Medicine,* 44: 681–92.

Cohen, S. and Williamson, G.M. (1991) Stress and infectious disease in humans, *Psychological Bulletin,* 109: 5–24.

Cohen, W.I. (1995) Family-oriented pediatric care, *Pediatric Clinics of North America,* 42(1): 11–19.

Cohen-Cole, S.A. (1991) *The Medical Interview: the Three Function Approach.* St Louis: Mosby.

Corney, R. (ed.) (1991) *Developing Communication and Counselling Skills in Medicine.* London: Tavistock/Routledge.

Covinsky, K.E., Goldman, L. and Cook, E.F. (1994) The impact of serious illness on patients' families, *Journal of the American Medical Association,* 272: 1839–44.

Craig, T.K.J. (1996) Adversity and depression, *International Review of Psychiatry,* 8: 341–53.

Cunningham-Burley, S. and Irvine S. (1987) 'And have you done anything so far?' An examination of lay treatment of children's symptoms, *British Medical Journal*, 295: 700–2.

Cunningham-Burley, S. and Maclean, U. (1987) Recognising and responding to children's symptoms: mothers' dilemmas, *Maternal and Child Health*, 12: 248–56.

Dalgleish, T. and Watts, F.N. (1990) Biases of attention and memory in disorders of anxiety and depression, *Clinical Psychology Review*, 10: 589–604.

Davenport, S., Goldberg, D. and Millar, T. (1987) How psychiatric disorders are missed during medical consultations, *Lancet*, 2: 439–41.

Davidoff, F. (1997) Time, *Annals of Internal Medicine*, 127: 483–5.

Del Mar, C. and Jewell, D. (1998) Tracking down the evidence, in C. Silagy and A. Haines (eds), *Evidence Based Practice in Primary Care*. London: British Medical Journal.

Eccles, M., Freemantle, N. and Mason, J. (1998) North of England evidence based guidelines development project: methods of developing guidelines, for efficient drug use in primary care, *British Medical Journal*, 316: 1232–35.

Egan, G. (1994) *The Skilled Helper*. Pacific Grove, CA: Brooks/Cole.

Eiser, C. (1990) *Chronic Childhood Disease*. Cambridge: Cambridge University Press.

Ekman, P., Friesen, W.V. and Ellsworth, P. (1972) *Emotions in the Human Face*. Elmsford, NY: Pergamon.

Elder, A. (1987) Moments of change, in A. Elder and O. Samuel (eds), *While I'm Here, Doctor*. London: Tavistock.

Elder, A. (1996) Enid Balint's contribution to general practice, *Psychoanalytic Psychotherapy*, 10: 101–8.

Elliott-Binns, C.P. (1986) An analysis of lay medicine: fifteen years later, *Journal of the Royal College of General Practitioners*, 36: 542–4.

Engel, G.L. (1977) The need for a new medical model: a challenge for biomedicine, *Science*, 196: 126–36.

Engel, G.L. (1980) The clinical application of the biopsychosocial model, *American Journal of Psychiatry*, 137: 535–44.

Enns, M.W. and Cox, B.J. (1997) Personality dimensions and depression: review and commentary, *Canadian Journal of Psychiatry*, 42: 274–84.

Evans, R.W. (1992) Some observations on whiplash injuries, *Neurologic Clinics*, 10: 975–97.

Fabrega, H. (1990) The concept of somatization as a cultural and historical product of western medicine, *Psychosomatic Medicine*, 52: 653–72.

Fahey, T. (1998) Applying the results of clinical trials to patients in general practice: perceived problems, strengths, assumptions, and challenges for the future, *British Journal of General Practice*, 48: 1173–8.

Freeling, P. and Harris, C.M. (1984) *The Doctor–Patient Relationship.* Edinburgh: Churchill Livingstone.

Freeman, G. and Hjortdahl, P. (1997) What future for continuity of care in general practice? *British Medical Journal,* 314: 1870–3.

Ferner, R.E. and Scott, D.K. (1994) Whatalotwegot – the messages in drug advertisements, *British Medical Journal,* 309: 1734–6.

France, R. and Robson, M. (1997) *Cognitive Behaviour Therapy in Primary Care.* London: Jessica Kingsley.

Frankel, R.M. (1989) Microanalysis and the medical encounter, in D.T. Helm, W.T. Anderson, A.J. Meehan and A.W. Rawls (eds), *The Interactional Order.* New York: Irvington.

Gale, J. and Marsden, P. (1983) *Medical Diagnosis.* Oxford: Oxford University Press.

Gask, L. (1995) Management in primary care, in C. Bass, M. Sharpe and R. Mayou (eds), *Medically Unexplained Symptoms.* Oxford: Oxford University Press.

Gardner, W.N. (1996) The pathophysiology of hyperventilation disorders, *Chest,* 109: 516–34.

Gerson, M., Grega, C.H. and Nathan-Virga, S. (1993) Three kinds of coping: families and inflammatory bowel disease, *Family Systems Medicine,* 11: 55–65.

Gibran, K. (1976) *The Prophet.* Bombay: Allied Publishers.

Gill, C. (1973) Types of interview in general practice: 'the flash', in E. Balint and J.S. Norell (eds), *Six Minutes for the Patient.* London: Tavistock.

Goldberg, D. and Bridges, K. (1988) Somatic presentations of psychiatric illness in primary care setting, *Journal of Psychosomatic Research,* 32: 137–44.

Goldberg, D. and Huxley, P. (1992) *Common Mental Disorders.* London: Routledge.

Goldberg, D., Gask, L. and O'Dowd, T. (1989) The treatment of somatization: teaching techniques of reattribution, *Journal of Psychosomatic Research,* 33: 689–95.

Goldberg, D.P., Jenkins, L., Millar, T. and Faragher, E.B. (1993) The ability of trainee general practitioners to identify psychological distress amongst their patients, *Psychological Medicine,* 23: 185–93.

Golden, G.A. and Brennan, M. (1995) Managing erotic feelings in the physician–patient relationship, *Canadian Medical Association Journal,* 153: 1241–5.

Greally, P., Cheng, K., Tanner, M.S. and Field, D.J. (1990) Children with croup presenting with scalds, *British Medical Journal,* 301: 113.

Greenhalgh, T. and Hurwitz, B. (1999) Narrative based medicine. Why study narrative? *British Medical Journal,* 318: 48–50.

Grol, R. (ed.) (1983) *To Heal or to Harm. The Prevention of Somatic Fixation in General Practice*. London: Royal College of General Practitioners.

Groves, J.E. (1978) Taking care of the hateful patient, *New England Journal of Medicine*, 298: 883–7.

Guthrie, E. (1996) Emotional disorder in chronic illness: psychotherapeutic interventions, *British Journal of Psychiatry*, 168: 265–73.

Halpern, J. (1993) Empathy: using resonance emotions in the service of curiosity, in H.M. Spiro, M.G.M. Curnen, E. Peschel and D. St James (eds), *Empathy and the Practice of Medicine*. New Haven, CT: Yale University Press.

Hampton, J.R., Harrison, M.J.G., Mitchell, J.R.A., Prichard, J.S. and Seymour, C. (1975) Relative contributions of history-taking, physical examination, and laboratory investigation to diagnosis and management of medical outpatients, *British Medical Journal*, 2: 486–9.

Hannay, D.R. (1979) *The Symptom Iceberg. A Study of Community Health*. London: Routledge & Kegan Paul.

Harrington, R., Whittaker, J., Shoebridge, P. and Campbell, F. (1998) Systematic review of efficacy of cognitive behaviour therapies in childhood and adolescent depressive disorder, *British Medical Journal*, 316: 1559–63.

Hart, J.T. (1994) *Feasible Socialism*. London: Socialist Health Association.

Hart, J.T., Thomas, C., Gibbons, B., Edwards, C., Hart, M., Jones, J., Jones, M. and Walton, P. (1991) Twenty five years of case finding and audit in a socially deprived community, *British Medical Journal*, 302: 1509–13.

Haynes, R.B., Sackett, D.L., Taylor, W., Gibson, E.S. and Johnson, A.L. (1978) Increased absenteeism from work after detection and labelling of hypertensive patients, *New England Journal of Medicine*, 299: 741–4.

Heath, I. (1995) *The Mystery of General Practice*. London: Nuffield Provincial Hospital Trust.

Heath, I. (1998) Doctors can do something about poverty, *British Medical Journal*, 316: 1456–7.

Helman, C.G. (1990) *Culture, Health and Illness*. Oxford: Butterworth-Heinemann.

Herman, J. (1989) The need for a transitional model: a challenge for biopsychosocial medicine? *Family Systems Medicine*, 7: 106–11.

Hobson, R.F. (1985) *Forms of Feeling*. London: Tavistock.

Hovenga, E., Kidd, M. and Cesnik, B. (1996) *Health Informatics: an Overview*. Melbourne: Churchill Livingstone.

Howie, J.G.R., Heaney, D.J. and Maxwell, M. (1997) *Measuring quality in general practice*. Occasional Paper 75. London: Royal College of General Practitioners.

Hunt, D.L., Haynes, R.B., Hanna, S.E. and Smith, K. (1998) Effects of computer-based clinical decision support systems on physician performance and patient outcomes, *Journal of the American Medical Association*, 280: 1339–46.

Jaber, R., Trilling, J.S. and Kelso, E.B. (1997) The circle of change: an approach to difficult clinical interactions, *Families, Systems and Health*, 15: 163–74.

Jenkins, R. and Clare, A. (1989) Women and mental illness, in P. Williams, G. Wilkinson and K. Rawnsley (eds) *The Scope of Epidemiological Psychiatry*. London: Routledge.

Johnson, T. (1984) *The Structure of Social Theory*. London: Macmillan.

Jorm, A.F. (1995) The epidemiology of depressive states in the elderly: implications for recognition, intervention and prevention, *Social Psychiatry and Psychiatric Epidemiology*, 30: 53–9.

Kagan, J. and Zentner, M. (1996) Early childhood predictors of adult psychopathology, *Harvard Review of Psychiatry*, 3: 341–50.

Kai, J. (1996) Parents' difficulties and information needs in coping with acute illness in preschool children: a qualitative study, *British Medical Journal*, 313: 987–90.

Kassirer, J.P. (1989) Diagnostic reasoning, *Annals of Internal Medicine*, 110: 893–900.

Katon, W. and Sullivan, M.D. (1990) Depression and chronic medical illness, *Journal of Clinical Psychiatry*, 51(6) (Suppl.): 3–11.

Kerr, C. (1998) Assessment of screening tests, in C. Kerr, R. Taylor and G. Heard (eds), *Handbook of Public Health Methods*. Sydney: McGraw-Hill.

Kerridge, I., Lowe, M. and Henry, D. (1998) Ethics and evidence based medicine, *British Medical Journal*, 316: 1151–3.

Kettell, J., Jones, R. and Lydeard, S. (1992) Reasons for consultation in irritable bowel syndrome: symptoms and patient characteristics, *British Journal of General Practice*, 42: 459–61.

Kleinman, A. (1988) *The Illness Narratives*. New York: Basic Books.

Korsch, B.M., Gozzi, E.K. and Francis, V. (1968) Gaps in doctor–patient communication. 1. Doctor–patient interaction and patient satisfaction, *Pediatrics*, 42: 855–71.

Korsch, B.M., Freemon, B. and Negrete, V.F. (1971) Practical implications of doctor–patient interaction analysis for pediatric practice, *American Journal of Disease in Childhood*, 121: 110–14.

Kriegsman, D.M.W., Penninx, B.W.J.H. and van Eijk, J.Th.M. (1995) A criterion-based literature survey of the relationship between family support and incidence and course of chronic disease in the elderly, *Family Systems Medicine*, 13: 39–68.

Laing, R.D. (1971) *The Politics of the Family*. London: Tavistock.

Lankton, S. (1980) *Practical Magic*. Cupertino, CA: Meta Publications.

Last, J.M. (1963) The iceberg: 'completing the clinical picture' in general practice, *Lancet*, 2: 28–31.

Last, J.M. (1994) The iceberg: 'completing the clinical picture' in general practice, in J. Ashton (ed.) *The Epidemiological Imagination*. Buckingham: Open University Press.

Launer, J. (1995) A social constructionist approach to family medicine, *Family Systems Medicine*, 13: 379–89.

Launer, J. and Lindsey, C. (1997) Training for systemic general practice: a new approach from the Tavistock Clinic, *British Journal of General Practice*, 47: 453–6.

Lefebvre, R.C., Hursey, K.G. and Carleton, R.A. (1988) Labelling of participants in high blood pressure screening programs: implications for blood cholesterol screenings, *Archives of Internal Medicine*, 148: 1993–7.

Levenstein, J.H., McCracken, E.C., McWhinney, I.R., Stewart, M.A. and Brown, J.B. (1986) The patient-centred clinical method. 1. A model for the doctor–patient interaction in family medicine, *Family Practice*, 3: 24–30.

Levinson, W., Roter, D.L., Mullooly, J.P., Dull, V.T. and Frankel, R.M. (1997) Physician–patient communication. The relationship with malpractice claims among primary care physicians and surgeons, *Journal of the American Medical Association*, 277: 553–9.

Ley, P. (1988) *Communicating with Patients*. London: Croom Helm.

Linfors, E.W. and Neelon, F.A. (1981) Interrogation and interview: strategies for obtaining clinical data, *Journal of the Royal College of General Practitioners*, 31: 426–8.

Little, M. (1995) *Humane Medicine*. Cambridge: Cambridge University Press.

Little, P., Williamson, I., Warner, G., Gould, C., Gantley, M. and Kinmonth, A.L. (1997) Open randomised trial of prescribing strategies in managing sore throat, *British Medical Journal*, 314: 722–7.

Lloyd, M. and Bor, R. (1996) *Communication Skills for Medicine*. Edinburgh: Churchill Livingstone.

MacLeod, C. (1991) Clinical anxiety and the selective encoding of threatening information, *International Review of Psychiatry*, 3: 279–92.

Malan, D.H. (1995) *Individual Psychotherapy and the Science of Psychodynamics*. Oxford: Butterworth-Heinemann.

Mathers, N., Jones, N. and Hannay, D. (1995) Heartsink patients: a study of their general practitioners, *British Journal of General Practice*, 45: 293–6.

Matthews, D.A., Suchman, A.L. and Branch, W.T. (1993) Making 'connexions': enhancing the therapeutic potential of patient–clinician relationships, *Annals of Internal Medicine*, 118: 973–7.

Mauksch, L.B. and Roesler, T. (1990) Expanding the context of the patient's explanatory model using circular questions, *Family Systems Medicine*, 8: 3–13.

Maxwell, P.R., Mendell, M.A. and Kumar, D. (1997) Irritable bowel syndrome, *Lancet*, 350: 1691–5.

McDaniel, S.H., Campbell, T. and Seaburn, D. (1989) Somatic fixation in patients and physicians: a biopsychosocial approach, *Family Systems Medicine*, 7: 5–16.

Mechanic, D. (1962) The concept of illness behaviour, *Journal of Chronic Disease*, 15: 189–94.

Morrell, D. (1998) As I recall, *British Medical Journal*, 317: 40–5.

Mullen, P.E., Martin, J.L., Anderson, J.C., Romans, S.E. and Herbison, G.P. (1993) Childhood sexual abuse and mental health in adult life, *British Journal of Psychiatry*, 163: 721–32.

Mumford, D.B. (1993) Somatization: a transcultural perspective, *International Review of Psychiatry*, 5: 231–42.

Mynors-Wallis, L. (1996) Problem-solving treatment: evidence for effectiveness and feasibility in primary care, *International Journal of Psychiatry in Medicine*, 26: 249–62.

Neighbour, R. (1987) *The Inner Consultation*. Lancaster: MTP Press.

Okri, B. (1996) *Birds of Heaven*. London: Phoenix.

Otten, M.W., Zaidi, A.A., Wroten, J.E., Witte, J.J. and Peterman, T.A. (1993) Changes in sexually transmitted disease rates after HIV testing and posttest counseling, Miami, 1988 to 1989, *American Journal of Public Health*, 83: 529–33.

Outhwaite, W. (1985) Hans-Georg Gadamer, in Q. Skinner (ed.) *The Return of Grand Theory in the Human Sciences*. Cambridge: Cambridge University Press.

Parkes, C.M. and Markus, A. (eds) (1998) *Coping with Loss*. London: BMJ Books.

Parsons, T. (1951) *The Social System*. London: Routledge & Kegan Paul.

Patterson, J.M. (1995) Promoting resilience in families experiencing stress, *Clinics of North America*, 42(1): 47–63.

Paykel, E.S. and Priest, R.G. (1992) Recognition and management of depression in general practice: consensus statement, *British Medical Journal*, 305: 1198–1202.

Pendleton, D., Schofield, T., Tate, P. and Havelock, P. (1984) *The Consultation: an Approach to Learning and Teaching*. Oxford: Oxford University Press.

Penninx, B.W.J.H., Kriegsman, D.M.W., van Eijk, J.Th.M., Boeke, A.J.P. and Deeg, D.J.H. (1996) Differential effect of social support on the course of chronic disease: a criteria-based literature study, *Families, Systems and Health*, 14: 223–44.

Peppiatt, R. (1992) Eliciting patients' views of the cause of their problem: a practical strategy for GPs, *Family Practice*, 9: 295–8.

Pilowsky, I. (1997) *Abnormal Illness Behaviour*. Chichester: Wiley.

Platt, F.W. (1995) *Conversation Repair*. Boston: Little, Brown.

Prochaska, J.O., DiClemente, C.C. and Norcross, J.C. (1992) In search of how people change, *American Psychologist*, 47: 1102–14.

Prochaska, J.O., Redding, C.A., Harlow, L.L., Rossi, J.S. and Velicer, W.F. (1994) The transtheoretical model of change and HIV prevention: a review, *Health Education Quarterly*, 21: 471–86.

Psathas, G. (1995) *Conversation Analysis*. Thousand Oaks, CA: Sage.

Qureshi, B. (1994) *Transcultural Medicine*. London: Libra Pharmaceuticals/Petrochemical Press.

Ramsey, P.G., Curtis, J.R., Paauw, D.S., Carline, J.D. and Wenrich, M.D. (1998) History-taking and preventive medicine skills among primary care physicians: an assessment using standardized patients, *American Journal of Medicine*, 104: 152–8.

Rees Lewis, J. (1994) Patient views on quality care in general practice: literature review, *Social Science and Medicine*, 39: 655–70.

Rogers, C.R. (1957) The necessary and sufficient conditions of therapeutic personality change, *Journal of Consulting Psychology*, 21: 95–103.

Rogers, C.R. (1975) Empathic: an unappreciated way of being, *Counseling Psychologist*, 5: 2–10.

Rose, G. (1992) *The Strategy of Preventive Medicine*. Oxford: Oxford University Press.

Roter, D.L., Stewart, M., Putnam, S.M., Lipkin, M., Stiles, W. and Inui, T.S. (1997) Communication patterns of primary care physicians, *Journal of the American Medical Association*, 277: 350–6.

Royal College of General Practitioners (1972) *The Future General Practitioner*. London: RCGP.

Rutter, P. (1995) *Sex in the Forbidden Zone*. London: HarperCollins.

Rycroft, C. (1995) *A Critical Dictionary of Psychoanalysis*. London: Penguin.

Sackett, D.L. (1992) A primer on the precision and accuracy of the clinical examination, *Journal of the American Medical Association*, 267: 2638–44.

Salinsky, J. (1987) Travelling hopefully, in A. Elder and O. Samuel (eds) *While I'm Here, Doctor*. London: Tavistock.

Salmon, P., Peters, S. and Stanley, I. (1999) Patients' perceptions of medical explanations for somatisation disorders: qualitative analysis, *British Medical Journal*, 318: 372–6.

Savage, R. and Armstrong, D. (1990) Effect of a general practitioner's consulting style on patient's satisfaction: a controlled study, *British Medical Journal*, 301: 968–70.

Schade, C.P., Jones, E.R. and Wittlin, B.J. (1998) A ten-year review of the validity and clinical utility of depression screening, *Psychiatric Services*, 49: 55–61.

Scheingold, L. (1988) Balint work in England: lessons for American family medicine, *Journal of Family Practice*, 26: 315–20.

Schild, P. and Herman, J. (1994) Somatic fixation revisited, *Family Systems Medicine*, 12: 31–6.

Scott, A.I.F. and Freeman, C.P.L. (1992) Edinburgh primary care depression study: treatment outcomes, patient satisfaction, and cost after 16 weeks, *British Medical Journal*, 304: 883–7.

Scott, J. (1996) Cognitive therapy of affective disorders: a review, *Journal of Affective Disorders*, 37: 1–11.

Shapiro, J. (1993) The use of narrative in the doctor–patient encounter, *Family Systems Medicine*, 11: 47–53.

Sifneos, P.E. (1996) Alexithymia: past and present, *American Journal of Psychiatry*, 153(7) (Suppl.): 137–42.

Silverman, J., Kurtz, S. and Draper, J. (1998) *Skills for Communicating with Patients*. London: Radcliffe.

Smith, G.R., Monson, R.A. and Ray, D.C. (1986) Psychiatric consultation in somatization disorder, *New England Journal of Medicine*, 314: 1407–13.

Smith, G.R., Rost, K. and Kashner, T.M. (1995) A trial of the effect of a standardised psychiatric consultation on health outcomes and costs in somatizing patients, *Archives of General Psychiatry*, 52: 238–43.

Smith, R.C. and Hoppe, R.B. (1991) The patient's story: integrating the patient- and physician-centred approaches to interviewing, *Annals of Internal Medicine*, 115: 470–7.

Sontag, S. (1990) *AIDS and its Metaphors*. London: Penguin.

Spiro, H.M. (1992) What is empathy and can it be taught? *Annals of Internal Medicine*, 116: 843–6.

Stewart, I. (1989) *Transactional Analysis Counselling in Action*. London: Sage.

Stewart, I. (1992) *Eric Berne*. London: Sage.

Stewart, M.A. (1995) Effective physician–patient communication and health outcomes: a review, *Canadian Medical Association Journal*, 152: 1423–33.

Stewart, M., Brown, J.B., Weston, W.W., McWhinney, I.R., McWilliam, C.L. and Freeman, T.R. (1995) *Patient-Centered Medicine*. Thousand Oaks, CA: Sage.

Storr, A. (1989) *Freud*. Oxford: Oxford University Press.

Stott, N.C.H. and Davis, R.H. (1979) The exceptional potential in each primary care consultation, *Journal of the Royal College of General Practitioners*, 29: 201–5.

Stott, N.C.H. and Pill, R.M. (1990) 'Advise yes, dictate no.' Patients' views on health promotion in the consultation, *Family Practice*, 7: 125–31.

Straus, J.L. and Cavanaugh, S. von A. (1996) Placebo effects. Issues for clinical practice in psychiatry and medicine, *Psychosomatics*, 37: 315–26.

Suchman, A.L., Markakis, K., Beckman, H.B. and Frankel, R. (1997) A model of empathic communication in the medical interview, *Journal of the American Medical Association*, 277: 678–82.

Sullivan, F. (1995) Intruders in the consultation, *Family Practice*, 12: 66–9.

Sullivan, F. M. and MacNaughton, R. J. (1996) Evidence in consultations: interpreted and individualised, *Lancet*, 348: 941–3.

ten Have, P. (1991) Talk and institution: a reconsideration of the 'asymmetry' of doctor–patient interaction, in D. Boden and D.H. Zimmerman (eds), *Talk and Social Structure*. Cambridge: Polity Press.

Thomas, K.B. (1987) General practice consultations: is there any point in being positive? *British Medical Journal*, 294: 1200–2.

Tuckett, D., Boulton, M., Olson, C. and Williams, A. (1985) *Meetings between Experts*. London: Tavistock.

Tymstra, T. and Bieleman, B. (1987) The psychosocial impact of mass screening for cardiovascular risk factors, *Family Practice*, 4: 287–90.

Ustun, T.B. and Sartorius, N. (1995) (eds) *Mental Illness in General Health Care*. Chichester: Wiley.

Usherwood, T.P. (1990) Responses to illness – implications for the clinician, *Journal of the Royal Society of Medicine* 83: 205–7.

Usherwood, T., Long, S. and Joesbury, H. (1997) The changing composition of primary health care teams, in P. Pearson and J. Spencer (eds), *Promoting Teamwork in Primary Care*. London: Arnold.

Van der Weijden, T. and Grol, R. (1998) Preventing recurrent coronary heart disease, *British Medical Journal*, 316: 1400–1.

Van Eijk, J., Grol, R., Huygens, F., Mesker, P., Mesker-Niesten, J., van Mierlo, G., Mokkink, H. and Smits, A. (1983) The family doctor and the prevention of somatic fixation, *Family Systems Medicine*, 1: 5–15.

Weingarten, K. and Worthen, M.E.W. (1997) A narrative approach to understanding the illness experiences of a mother and daughter, *Families, Systems and Health*, 15: 41–54.

Williams, J.W. and Simel, D.L. (1992) Does this patient have ascites? *Journal of the American Medical Association*, 267: 2645–8.

Williams, P.R. (1989) *Family Problems*. Oxford: Oxford University Press.

Wilson, J. and Jungner, G. (1968) *Principles and Practices of Screening for Disease*. WHO Public Health Paper, No. 34. Geneva: World Health Organization.

World Health Organization (1992) *The ICD-10 Classification of Mental and Behavioural Disorders: Clinical Descriptions and Diagnostic Guidelines.* Geneva: WHO.

World Health Organization (1993) *The ICD-10 Classification of Mental and Behavioural Disorders: Diagnostic Criteria for Research.* Geneva: WHO.

Zigmond, D. (1978) When Balinting is mind-rape, *Update*, 16: 1123–6.

Zola, I.K. (1966) Culture and symptoms: an analysis of patients' presenting complaints, *American Sociological Review*, 31: 615–30.

Zola, I.K. (1973) Pathways to the doctor: from person to patient, *Social Science and Medicine*, 7: 677–89.

Index

COUNSELLING IN MEDICAL SETTINGS

Patricia East

Fundamental changes in the management and delivery of health and community care have resulted from recent government initiatives. At the same time the complex personal relationship between physical, social, environmental and emotional aspects of illness is increasingly being recognized in medical settings. Many claims have been made to justify an expansion of counselling in medical settings as a response to these changes, not only as a supportive therapeutic experience but also as a healing process in its own right. This timely book describes the emergence and growth of counselling in medical settings and examines the issues surrounding its incorporation into this context. Written in a clear accessible style it provides not only a broad overview of counselling and counselling skills but also focuses on specific issues pertinent to counsellors from a wide variety of medical backgrounds. Patricia East's account of counselling in medical settings and the meaning of illness for individuals is enlivened by the extensive use of examples and case material from practitioners.

Contents
The development of counselling in medical settings – Counselling in medical settings – The practice of counselling in medical settings – Specific issues in counselling in medical settings – Professional relationships in counselling in medical settings – A critique of counselling in medical settings – References – Index.

168pp   0 335 19241 6 (Paperback)

PRIMARY CARE
MAKING CONNECTIONS

Noel Boaden

- How should the professional career in primary care be seen in light of the intentions for a primary care-led NHS and what changes does this suggest in professional education?
- How might primary care be organized to provide the right context for such professional careers and a framework which can facilitate the formal politics and public participation which give it legitimacy?

This book looks at primary care in a broad way which goes beyond the idea that it is only about general practice. It explores the linkages involved in that extended view through an examination of the history of development in healthcare and through the application of a systems analysis to that process.

In light of that discussion it then examines the current organization and management of primary care and the fragmented professional staffing in relation to the demands of a primary care-led NHS. These chapters lead on to consideration of new forms of organization in primary care and the development of the professions involved and their education and training. Recommendations are made about both aspects as a framework for a consideration of the politics of primary care both institutionally and in relation to emerging ideas about citizen participation.

Contents

176pp   0 335 19748 5 (Paperback)   0 335 19749 3 (Hardback)

MEDICAL MISHAPS
PIECES OF THE PUZZLE

**Marilynn M. Rosenthal, Linda Mulcahy and
Sally Lloyd-Bostock**

> I believe that this important collection will very quickly be-
> come a key text in this area. It should be a must for students,
> researchs and health care professionals.
> Jonathan Gabe, Royal Holloway, University of London.

This book explores what we know about the incidence, causes
and aftermath of medical mishaps. Increasingly the medical pro-
fession is being expected to review the performance of doctors
more rigorously and systematically and to adopt proactive
approaches to the management of risk. Little is known about how
often medical mishaps occur, the proportion which are prevent-
able and the impact of the mishap on those involved. Contribu-
tors to this volume are all experts in their field who can reveal
something about medical mishap puzzles from a UK and international perspective. Medical mishaps are traced from their genesis
and cause through to the impact they have on doctors, patients,
managers, educators and those respeonsible for the resolution of
complaints and medical negligence disputes arising from them.
This volume is unique in bringing together a number of different
voices. The contributions are multi-disciplinary and report both
empirical studies of these phenomena as well as the experiences
of those who have to deal with medical mishaps on a day-to-day
basis.

Contents
*Part One: Mapping and understanding medical mishaps – Part Two:
International perspectives – Part Three: The escalation and mitigation of
mishaps – Part Four: Views from the coalface: The doctor's perspective –
Views from the coalface: The manager's perspective – Views from the
coalface: The patient's perspective – Index.*

288pp   0 335 20258 6 (Paperback)   0 335 20259 4 (Hardback)